RESOUNDING ACCLAIM FOR
SAVE YOUR HEARING NOW

"There is no question that Dr. Seidman's four-step method of good nutrition, exercise, and noise protection, combined with vitamin supplementation, will improve the hearing health of all those who follow his prescription. I congratulate Dr. Seidman for bringing this important information to the general public."

—LAWRENCE R. LUSTIG, MD, associate professor, Department of Otolaryngology-Head and Neck Surgery, University of California San Francisco

"I wish I had written this book myself! It is accurate, timely, and forward-looking. Dr. Seidman is among the leaders in the treatment of hearing loss with nutrition and supplementation. I heartily endorse these principles and use them for myself and my patients."

—CHARLES I. BERLIN, PhD, Kenneth and Frances Barnes Bullington Professor of Hearing Science, Louisiana State University Health Sciences Center, Department of Otolaryngology-Head and Neck Surgery

"SAVE YOUR HEARING NOW explains the value of alternative methods for treating hearing impairment through antioxidants and nutrition . . . Comprehensive and well written, it will be of great interest to all who suffer from hearing loss."

—HOWARD P. HOUSE, MD, for and founder, House

SAVE YOUR
HEARING
NOW

THE REVOLUTIONARY PROGRAM
THAT CAN PREVENT AND MAY
EVEN REVERSE HEARING LOSS

MICHAEL D. SEIDMAN, MD, FACS
Director of Otologic/Neurotologic Surgery
and Otolaryngology Research,
Henry Ford Health Systems
AND MARIE MONEYSMITH

WARNER
WELLNESS

NEW YORK   BOSTON

you purchase this book without a cover you should be aware that this book may have been stolen property and reported as "unsold and destroyed" to the publisher. In such case neither the author nor the publisher has received any payment for this "stripped book."

This book is not intended as a substitute for medical advice of physicians. The reader should regularly consult a physician in all matters relating to his or her health, and particularly in respect of any symptoms that may require diagnosis or medical attention.

Copyright © 2006 by Michael D. Seidman, MD, FACS, and Marie Moneysmith
All rights reserved. Except as permitted under the U.S. Copyright Act of 1976, no part of this publication may be reproduced, distributed, or transmitted in any form or by any means, or stored in a database or retrieval system, without the prior written permission of the publisher.

Book design and text composition by L&G McRee

Ear diagram on page 15 by Jay Knipstein.

Warner Wellness
Hachette Book Group USA
237 Park Avenue
New York, NY 10169
Visit our Web site at www.HachetteBookGroupUSA.com

Printed in the United States of America

Originally published in hardcover by Warner Books.
First Trade Edition: May 2007

10 9 8 7 6 5 4 3 2 1

Warner Wellness is a trademark of Time Warner Inc. or an affiliated company. Used under license by Hachette Book Group USA, which is not affiliated with Time Warner Inc.

The Library of Congress has cataloged the hardcover edition as follows:

Seidman, Michael D.
    Save your hearing now : the revolutionary program that can prevent and may even reverse hearing loss / Michael D. Seidman and Marie Moneysmith.
        p. cm.
    Includes index.
    ISBN-13: 978-0-446-57843-1
    ISBN-10: 0-446-57843-6
    1. Deafness—Popular works. 2. Deafness—Prevention—Popular works.
I. Moneysmith, Marie. II. Title.
    RF291.35.S43 2006
    617. 8—dc22

                                                    2005034304

ISBN-13: 978-0-446-69620-3 (pbk.)
ISBN-10: 0-446-69620-X (pbk.)

ACKNOWLEDGMENTS

To give thanks and appreciation to my teachers, co-workers, and my patients, (who are always the best teachers) would take a whole extra book. Dozens of people have made this book possible, including the many wonderful physicians, residents, and mentors I have learned from over the years. The short list includes Dr. Richard Nichols, Dr. Herbert Silverstein, Dr. Malcolm Graham, Dr. Michael Benninger, and the late Dr. John Kemink, but there are so many others. Sincere thanks also to my close personal scientific colleagues that I have had the privilege of learning from and collaborating with over the past twenty years, including Fred Nuttall, PhD, Wayne Quirk, PhD, Josef Miller, PhD, and Jochen Schacht, PhD.

To Bill Gates, whose business acumen and his ability to grow his product/expertise globally have been a huge inspiration. I have always been overwhelmed by his ability and his commitment to give back to those who are less fortunate. He is truly an exceptional role model.

Evan Weiner, a brilliant businessman, has always provided me with unbelievable encouragement to pursue my nutritional interests. I am also grateful to Marti Felder, PA, who helps to make my work life a pleasure.

I owe a great deal to Chris Tomasino, a superlative agent who shepherded this project through the publishing world with skill and good humor; to Marie Moneysmith, who helped articulate the many years of science and clinical practice relevant to this book; and to Diana Baroni, the editor writers dream of but seldom find.

I am eternally grateful for the support of my family—my wife, Lynn, in particular, as well as our three very special children, Jake, Marlee, and Kevin—who allow me to understand the meaning of the words *pride*, *love*, and *affection*. I am truly blessed. Many thanks to my parents, Mel and Rita Seidman, who always said: You can do and be whatever you want, as long as you never quit, are true to your morals and ethics, and do the right thing. They have made me believe that anything is possible. I am grateful, too, to my wife's parents, Robert and Roberta Gaberman, who have welcomed me into their family and are truly the best in-laws ever. I would not be here today without their love and support, as well as the encouragement of my brother, Steve, and sister, Amy.

Lastly, to all of you who have taken the time to read this book and pass it on to your friends and family. The bottom line is that we *can* make a difference, and I would like to start with you.

CONTENTS

INTRODUCTION

What do actors Halle Berry, Rob Lowe, Sylvester Stallone, and Paul Newman have in common with former president Bill Clinton, golf legend Arnold Palmer, and rockers Sting, Pete Townshend, and Ozzy Osbourne? Surprising as it may seem, the answer is hearing loss. And they are far from alone. Half of the nearly 76 million baby boomers (individuals between forty and fifty-nine years old) in the United States say they are dealing with some degree of hearing loss. That's a 238 percent increase since 1990, when hearing problems affected only 20 percent of this group.

Hearing loss is on the brink of becoming a major health issue, rivaling the obesity epidemic in sheer numbers. In the United States, the baby boomers hold first place, with more than 30 million sufferers. Second place goes to the 9 million hearing-impaired individuals over the age of sixty-five. One-third of these seniors live with hearing loss so severe it interferes with daily life. Given the current rate of increase in the elderly segment of the population, by 2050 the number of hearing-impaired people in this country will be growing faster than the total population of the United States.

Unfortunately, you don't have to be middle-aged or elderly to experience hearing loss. A 1998 study, reported in the *Journal of the American Medical Association* (*JAMA*), concluded that nearly 15 percent of children between the ages of five and nineteen have hearing difficulties. That translates into about 2 million hearing-impaired youngsters, says Hearing Alliance of America. And hearing loss is becoming increasingly common among younger people. In fact, a National Health Interview Survey found that hearing difficulties increased by almost 20 percent among eighteen- to forty-four-year-olds between 1971 and 1990.

Problems with hearing can be difficult to detect, especially in the early stages. In certain situations, such as a one-on-one conversation in a quiet place, there may be no apparent symptoms. Yet at other times—in a crowded restaurant filled with background noises, for example—it's a struggle to hear what is being said by dinner companions. Certainly, bad acoustics can be at least partly to blame. But when an individual frequently has to ask people to repeat themselves, often misunderstands conversations, or tends to turn up the television volume, it could be due to hearing loss.

As I will explain, hearing is possible because of the intricate and sophisticated auditory system, brilliant in many ways. Of course, sophisticated machines are notoriously sensitive and prone to breaking down. And as anyone who has become frustrated with a malfunctioning computer knows, the experience can be maddening. The same is true of the auditory system. When it is working well, we send and receive information effortlessly, without even pausing to marvel at the wonders of the process. But when things go wrong, an ordinary conversation turns into an exercise in frustration and misunderstanding. Sometimes the result is simply embarrassing or silly enough to be laughed off, but there are occasions when the consequences of not hearing correctly can be serious. Imagine what might happen if a doctor's instructions, for example, are not heard properly.

The traditional solution to hearing problems is a hearing aid. While these devices have improved greatly in recent years, they still have shortcomings, which we will look at later. Meanwhile, newer technological breakthroughs, such as cochlear implants, have achieved such miraculous results that they are changing the lives of many individuals whose hearing loss was beyond the help of hearing aids. But with price tags starting at $50,000, cochlear implants are simply out of reach for many people.

More than twenty years ago, I began studying hearing loss, both with my patients and in the laboratory. While there are hearing devices to help the impaired, there seems to be less research and focus on the preventative and treatment aspects of hearing loss. In theory, it seemed that if we could identify the cause of the problem, we could find a way to prevent or reverse it. My purpose was to identify a natural means of repairing the damage that caused common hearing loss. And after a great deal of research—funded by more than $1.5 million in research grants from the National Institutes of Health and other respected organizations—I firmly believe that it is now possible. And I now want to share it with you in *Save Your Hearing Now*.

The research my colleagues and I have done, which has been thoroughly reviewed by other experts and published in leading medical journals, clearly demonstrates that we can slow the progression of—and in some cases, reverse—hearing loss with natural substances found in food and supplements. As the growth of alternative medicine demonstrates, a healthful diet and supplemental nutrients are tremendously powerful allies for many individuals, especially those who have not found solutions or remedies in conventional medicine. As you will see, the medical profession is now recognizing that such lifestyle choices as what you have for dinner and which vitamins you do (or don't) take are directly connected to how well the body performs a wide range of functions, and hearing is no exception. I have no doubt that you can protect hearing and slow hearing loss by taking advantage of the powerful foods and nutrients in this program.

In addition, you can support and amplify the effects of those compounds with other lifestyle changes detailed in the Save Your Hearing Now Program. I will explain why specific elements of the program are included, how they work to improve and protect hearing, and help you create an individualized regimen that is both effective and easy to live with.

Since hearing is highly localized, at first glance it may seem odd to be concerned with anything other than the ears. From a medical standpoint, however, it's important to understand that the human body works best when all the parts are cared for and kept in good working order. While much of the medical profession today is specialized and focused on particular aspects of health, we need to remember that every element in the body is part of the whole. And for this reason, I believe in a holistic approach to treating hearing loss that rebuilds and defends all of our cells, with particular emphasis on those in our auditory system.

Even if you are not suffering from age-related hearing loss, however, there are still reasons to read this book. One, this book offers a preventative strategy using diet and nutrients to not only improve your hearing but also reduce the likelihood of experiencing hearing loss. A second reason is the widespread, serious, but seldom-addressed phenomenon of noise pollution, the subject of a presentation I made before Congress in 2004. The planet we live on is noisier than it has ever been, at least since human habitation began. Our ears were not designed to cope with the incessant din that surrounds many of us, and for more than thirty years, there has been a growing body of scientific research showing that noise—even if it is not very loud—takes a toll on the hearing, health, and emotions of adults and children alike.

If the bad news is that noise is everywhere, that aging is a given, and that both can harm your hearing and your health, the good news is that now you can do something about it. Actually, there's a great deal you can do about it. The process begins by reading this book and following the recommendations in the Save Your Hearing Now Program, whether you have hearing loss or are seeking to prevent it.

In this book, I will present the latest scientific findings on hearing loss—what causes it, how it can be prevented, and treatment that works. The first section of the book details the intricate structure of the ears and the process of hearing, as well as various factors that can interfere with or promote our hearing. In the second section, I will present the latest groundbreaking research on the effects of diet, physical fitness, antioxidants, and supplements on hearing, and guide you through methods for applying each element for optimal auditory health. Finally, I will offer further preventative measures to preserve your hearing, as well as alternative therapies for specific hearing-related problems. All will combine to create an overall program that can prevent and may even reverse hearing loss. This valuable collection of research, information, and recommondations can be used as an aid in your quest for optimal hearing health.

SAVE YOUR
HEARING
NOW

((1))

THE MANY TOLLS OF HEARING LOSS

"I like your watch. What kind is it?"
"About quarter to three."

"The chicken looks good. Do you want white meat or thighs?"
"Oh, no fries for me, thanks."

"The lawyer said he can see you tomorrow. Is three okay?"
"Sure . . . but why is it free?"

Most of us have had little misunderstandings when words weren't heard correctly. But when these incidents become a regular part of the day, hearing loss could be to blame. The best way to determine how well hearing is working is by having an evaluation by a hearing professional—starting with an otolaryngologist/head and neck surgeon (also known as an ear, nose, and throat doctor, or ENT) and an audiologist. But here are a few signs that may help determine whether it's time to make that appointment:

- People often have to repeat themselves when speaking to you, or you think that others are mumbling when they speak.
- You find yourself straining to hear conversations in public places, especially when there is background noise.
- When the television volume or music is loud enough for you to hear comfortably, it is too loud for others in the room.
- Errors have occurred because information or instructions were not heard correctly.
- Telephone conversations are difficult because it's hard to hear the other party.
- You fail to hear the doorbell, kitchen timer, alarm clock, or other appliance.

Today, more people than ever before are dealing with hearing loss. In fact, the numbers are staggering—more than 30 million baby boomers, another 9 million seniors, and some 2 million young people. Worldwide, the numbers soar to 500 million—including 70 million Europeans—making hearing loss the number one disability in the world.

Hearing's Two Worst Enemies: Aging and Noise

The epidemic levels of hearing loss can be explained partially by the fact that we are living longer and aging takes a toll on hearing. But there is a second, more dangerous hearing enemy at work, too—noise. If you think about the world we live in, this steep increase in hearing loss is not surprising. Each and every day, the average person is assaulted by an extraordinary amount of noise. In many cases, the sources are convenience devices and appliances we depend on—hair dryers, garbage disposals, sound-producing toys, personal music players, lawn mowers, and vacuum cleaners, to name only a few.

Sound researchers have measured the intensity of many every-day noises and made some surprising conclusions. For example:

- Young people often drive cars with stereo systems that can be as noisy as a jet during takeoff.
- Movie sound tracks blasting from theaters' multispeaker systems rival the sound levels of power saws.
- The roar of a garbage disposal is nearly as earsplitting as a tractor engine.
- Hair dryers can blow away sandblasters, in terms of volume.
- The ear-piercing sounds made by certain children's toys are just about off the charts, sometimes matching air-raid sirens in intensity.
- An evening in a karaoke bar can cost a lot in terms of hearing. The combined effects of singing and music can go well above 95 decibels (dB).
- If you're going to the gym, choose your aerobics classes carefully—and get a spot as far from the speakers as possible. Noise levels from a gym's sound system frequently hit the 90+ dB range.

COMMON SOUNDS IN DECIBELS

15	The average threshold of human hearing (although some people can hear sounds in the 0 to 15 dB range)
20	The sound of a human whisper
50–60	Normal conversation
75	A typical vacuum cleaner
85–90	The point at which hearing damage begins (e.g., a hair dryer or a quiet lawn mower)
100	Power saw
120	Snowmobile engine, jackhammer, chain saw
135	A jet on takeoff, amplified music
140	Gunshot, emergency sirens, threshold of noise-induced pain

Since many tools and toys are commonplace, we tend to take the constant din for granted. In fact, we are so accustomed to noise that silence has become suspicious. Reportedly, back in the 1940s, a silent vacuum cleaner, equipped with an efficient but noiseless induction motor, failed to impress buyers; no one believed that a suction device could work without making noise.

NOISE IN THE WORKPLACE

Work-related noise is the leading occupational disease, and experts estimate that about 30 million Americans are exposed to toxic noise levels at work. Furthermore, 10 million people have hearing loss caused by excessive noise at work, according to the Deafness Research Foundation (DRF; www.drf.org).

Even the quiet country life is hard to find, thanks to noise from farm machinery. And as a recent Minnesota survey found, farmers are feeling the effects. Fully two-thirds of those queried not long ago had moderate or significant hearing loss.

Bottom line: Hearing's greatest enemy is damage caused by aging. But today, noise is a close second, increasing the likelihood that millions of people will be forced to cope with impaired hearing *before middle age even begins.*

Since good hearing is essential to the learning process, children and young people are particularly affected by hearing difficulties. Unfortunately, many children with poor hearing are misdiagnosed as having learning disabilities. The hearing problems are never identified or corrected, leading to a vicious cycle with potentially serious complications, including social problems, unwarranted disciplinary actions, and major emotional difficulties.

Frequently, those children whose hearing loss is discovered and corrected don't fare much better, because wearing hearing aids sets them apart from their peers at a time when being different is difficult at best. Says the mother of a nine-year-old boy who suffers from hearing loss: "Having hearing aids at such an early age is a tremendous problem. Kids are so mean about his need for help. He's a bright, normal child except for his hearing, and they treat him like he's from another planet."

The Hidden Costs of Hearing Loss

Clearly, hearing loss is more than an inconvenience. Like all ailments, difficulties with hearing take a personal and public toll. But while experts have calculated the costs to society of various health concerns, such as heart disease, obesity, and diabetes, no one tallies the economic costs of hearing loss. If we added up hearing-loss-related costs—errors made, the time spent correcting them, faulty products that have to be discarded and redone, information that never reaches the right destination, all creating delays, additional expenditures, overtime charges, and so on—it's safe to assume that the grand total would easily reach billions of dollars every year. The U.S. Navy alone estimates its own costs related to noise-induced hearing loss at approximately $1 billion annually, a mind-numbing figure, and further proof that this is a problem that has reached epidemic proportions.

While we may never know exactly how much money hearing loss is leaching from our economy, we do know a few things:

- According to an in-depth study published in the *International Journal of Technology Assessment in Health Care 2000,* between 500,000 and 750,000 Americans suffer from severe to profound hearing loss, which costs society nearly $300,000 per person during each individual's life. The grand total is well into the trillions of dollars.
- The earlier hearing loss is diagnosed, the more costly it is. Expenditures for social services, specialized education, and treatment of a hearing-impaired child can easily run as high as $1 million over that child's lifetime.
- Hearing difficulty is the second most common complaint (after arthritis) reported to doctors by elderly patients.
- It has been estimated that nearly 13 percent of all soldiers being sent home from Operation Iraqi Freedom are suffering from hearing-related trauma. Furthermore, about one-fourth of America's combat personnel develop significant hearing loss, and the condition is now one of the top ten disabilities for Veterans Affairs.

As serious as the economic cost of hearing loss may be, it cannot compete with the emotional toll. People who live with diminished hearing and those who share their lives—as spouses and partners, co-workers, friends, relatives, clients, and neighbors—consider hearing loss emotionally devastating.

THE PEACE AND QUIET MOVEMENT

The importance of maintaining a quiet community is becoming recognized all over the country. Neighbors of the Michigan State Fairgrounds near Detroit, for example, successfully fought plans for an Indy-style auto racing track that would have funneled millions of dollars into the area. Why? They were opposed to the noise that would have been generated by the race cars and added traffic to the area.

Similarly, in New York City, where noise is a serious problem, city officials are cracking down on noise polluters with a new noise code, designed to incorporate high-tech acoustic technology and update sections of the existing code.

Compromising Careers

For more than a decade, Carren Stika, Ph.D., of National University in La Jolla, California, has studied the psychosocial impact of hearing loss. One of her recent research projects examines how hearing loss affects work and career. Preliminary findings show about one-third of those with hearing difficulties feel incompetent or stressed at work, yet almost 40 percent of these individuals say they would "rarely" or "almost never" ask for an adjustment or accommodation because of it. Why? Because they're embarrassed to admit that they don't hear well.

With hearing loss, carrying on a conversation turns into an exercise in frustration. Business meetings, seminars, conferences, and phone calls become major sources of stress. Misunderstanding directions can be disastrous. Even lunch in a busy restaurant is more than some people with hearing problems can endure.

A fifty-two-year-old advertising copywriter, for example, remembers a particularly painful experience, when she was one of the final contenders for a staff job at a major advertising agency. The human resources director invited her to lunch with a few people from the company. "At first, every-thing was great," she says. "But as the restaurant started filling up, it became harder and harder for me to hear the people sitting on the other side of the table.

"I knew one of the women slightly and knew that her hus-band had just had an operation, so I asked how he was. I thought she said, 'The doctor said he's doing fine,' and I told her that was excellent and I was very glad to hear it. Everyone turned and looked at me like I was out of my mind. Finally, the woman next to me said, 'I think you misunderstood. The doctor said her husband is going blind.'

"Of course, I apologized profusely. But I was mortified. I didn't talk again during lunch, and I didn't get the job, either."

Losing Hearing, Losing Friends

While careers can be compromised by hearing loss, leisure ac-tivities are affected by an inability to hear, too. Nearly all en-tertainment relies on hearing, but you can't turn up the volume at plays, movie theaters, or concerts. Is it any surprise that people with hearing loss often prefer isolation to strug-gling through social functions and entertainment venues out-side the home?

Ted and his wife, Jean, had been regular churchgoers until Jean's hearing began to deteriorate. At first, she claimed her re-luctance to go out was because the winter weather had made driving too dangerous. But when spring arrived, she was forced to admit that the real reason she didn't want to attend services any longer was that she couldn't hear the sermon or manage conversations during the social hour afterward. As re-tirees in a small town with no family nearby, Ted and Jean had limited social opportunities to begin with. Eliminating church-going from their week left them virtually isolated and out of touch with a group of people they had enjoyed.

I heard Ted and Jean's story from Jean's brother, Bill. He came to see me because his wife had fallen down the basement stairs recently and sprained her ankle, but he hadn't heard her cries for help because the radio volume had been so loud. That was all the motivation Bill needed to do something about his hearing, which had been steadily declining. After a long bout with the flu, he felt his hearing had taken a serious hit. "What if my wife had a heart attack or who knows what and I didn't hear her?" he explained. "Plus, I don't want to end up like my sister and brother-in-law, sitting in the house with the TV blasting all day because they can't have a conversation with anyone."

After several months on the Save Your Hearing Now Program, Bill's hearing stabilized, and he was so encouraged that he recommended it to Jean and Ted. "I hope they follow through on it," Bill said. "If they don't do something soon, I'm afraid they'll become completely deaf in a few years."

Needless to say, individuals with hearing loss aren't the only ones who suffer. Family members, friends, and co-workers are frustrated, too, as they are forced to repeat themselves, deal with uncomfortably loud televisions and radios, and worry about whether important information was heard or not. "I was so tired of repeating myself whenever I spoke to my husband that I began avoiding conversations with him," recalls one woman whose husband's hearing deteriorated sharply when he was in his late fifties. "He thought I was angry, but I just couldn't take it anymore."

Or the opposite problem may occur. Some individuals with hearing loss worry about talking too loudly and end up speaking so softly it's difficult to hear them, creating even more frustration for those around them.

With today's longer life spans and our increasingly noisy world, everyone's hearing is at risk. So the sooner we begin to preserve our hearing and work at correcting hearing loss, the better. Unfortunately for some, hearing devices are necessary. Major strides in technology have made these devices smaller and more sophisticated than ever before, but they are still not stylish or chic (like glasses can be, for instance), and there is definitely a stigma attached to wearing them. (From my perspective, I find the attitude that hearing aids are embarrassing completely inappropriate. Hearing aids are immensely helpful for people with hearing difficulties, and no one should feel ashamed about correcting the problem by wearing one.) Fortunately for many hearing loss sufferers—even some of the ones who have or may need hearing devices—there are now proven methods of protecting and even rehabilitating your hearing. Whether you are young or old, have hearing loss or are worried about developing it, this program is for you.

The Save Your Hearing Now Program incorporates antioxidant and mitochondrial-enhancing supplements and foods that provide vitally important nutrients that protect and rejuvenate cells throughout the body, as well as physical activity and other lifestyle measures that bolster their effects. Hundreds of studies have shown that such a treatment regimen can have a profound effect on the damage caused by aging, pollution, poor diet, sedentary lifestyle, and stress. Far too few of us—including those who eat carefully—are getting sufficient quantities of the right substances or physical activity, but the Save Your Hearing Now Program is designed to help you incorporate all the necessary nutrients and lifestyle changes in order to obtain optimal—or much-improved— hearing health. Hundreds of patients have experienced significant improvements in their hearing with this easy, inexpensive approach, which is equally effective for all age groups. The dramatic results that are possible with this program are truly creating a revolution in the treatment of hearing loss. But before we get into the details of the Save Your Hearing Now Program, let's take an in-depth look at how the amazing process of hearing works.

((**2**))

HOW HEARING HAPPENS

Ears are marvels of engineering. These compact, highly complex organs relay a constant stream of information to the brain. There, sounds are interpreted to determine an appropriate reaction. Although some animals' hearing is more sensitive than ours, a normal, healthy human ear processes a fairly wide range of sounds, and does so with incredible efficiency and speed.

In order to fully understand how hearing loss can be repaired or prevented, it's important to know how hearing works in the first place. In this chapter, we will look at the basic elements of the ear and discover how this small, underrated organ is able to translate the vibrations called sound into a wide range of useful information. To do that, I will occasionally delve into technical detail that may seem overwhelming at first. But if you stay with me, you will learn about the remarkable process of hearing, so you can better understand what causes hearing loss and how it can be prevented and corrected.

From the Outside In

When it comes to hearing, the outer, visible part of the ear is only the tip of the iceberg. The exterior portion of the ear, or outer ear, is called the *auricle,* which comes from the Latin word for ear, *auricula.* It is also sometimes referred to as the *pinna,* or "feather" in Latin. This part of the ear is made of skin and cartilage, which makes it strong and flexible at the same time.

Technically speaking, we do not hear with the auricle. The swirling, curved structure of this part of the ear is designed to capture sounds and send them further inside the organ. In a sense, the auricle is simply a funnel. Its primary function is to gather and relay all the random sounds occurring in the environment, without evaluating or filtering. The fact that we have two ears has nothing to do with stereo capability; instead, it allows the brain to determine which side of the body a sound is coming from. If the waves originate from a source on the left, they arrive at the left ear a microsecond before entering the right ear. This may not seem particularly important. But patients who lose hearing in only one ear often say that not being able to determine the source of a sound can be very disturbing—and in some situations, even dangerous—since they can't tell, for example, if that car horn that is honking is on the right or the left.

Sound travels in waves that are produced by air particle movement. A simple example is the quiet swishing sound heard when you wave a fan back and forth. Larger, heavier objects make louder noises when they move. Various factors influence how loud a sound is, including the size of the object, the speed at which it is moving, and its proximity to the ear. The sound of a piano being played is much louder, for example, to the person who is playing it than to someone in the next room.

Sound waves that reach the auricle move into a short tube (about one inch in length and one-quarter inch in diameter) known as the *ear canal*. One of the ear canal's duties is to convey sound vibrations further into the ear. It is also responsible for producing earwax, which is not really "wax" at all but a secretion known as *cerumen,* created by special glands. Although it may seem like a nuisance, earwax has a purpose: keeping harmful substances from reaching the ear's interior. Dust and dirt, for example, become stuck in earwax so they cannot move any further into the ear canal, and the wax itself is comprised of antibacterial chemicals that ward off infections. Earwax also provides a bit of waterproofing for the interior portion of the ear.

THE RIGHT WAY TO CLEAN EARS

Although the eardrum consists of three layers of skin, it is quite delicate and can be punctured easily. Even something fairly soft, like a cotton swab, can perforate the eardrum. So when patients ask how to clean their ears, here is my answer. Do not put anything smaller than your elbow in your ears—ever! And yes, that includes cotton swabs. Since they are similar in diameter to the ear canal, swabs look like the perfect cleaning tool. And if you put a cotton swab in your ear canal, you will see wax on the end of it. Unfortunately, what you *can't* see is that you have just packed far more wax *into* the ear, very close to the eardrum. About once a month, I have to repair eardrums ruptured by cotton swabs, keys, hairpins, and other objects.

So how can ears be safely cleaned? Generally speaking, the ears are self-cleaning. Wax is slowly swept to the outer canal, and from there it can be wiped gently away with a washcloth and finger. (Yes, a finger is smaller than an elbow—you caught me there—but this method is still pretty safe.)

If this is not satisfactory, mix a little hot tap water with cool (room temperature) hydrogen peroxide—about half and half. Test a few drops of the mixture on the inside of your wrist to make sure it is about body temperature. Then use an eyedropper to fill one ear canal with this solution. Tip your head to the opposite side, so the solution stays inside the canal, and stay in this position for one or two minutes. Then tip your head back to the other side, so the excess solution can trickle out. Repeat the process in the other ear. This can be done once a month, if necessary.

A word of caution about this method: Some people lose their equilibrium or become dizzy when liquid that is warmer or colder than the body enters the ear canal. This is a perfectly normal response. If you experience dizziness or light-headedness, try sitting down or have someone stand at your side to help you stay upright while the solution is in the ear canal. The feeling is usually temporary, and equilibrium is restored when the liquid drains out.

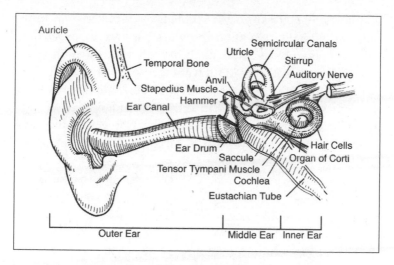

Figure 1: **The anatomy of the ear**

Sounds Good

After sound waves travel through the ear canal, they arrive at the eardrum, or *tympanic membrane*. The eardrum lives up to its name, since it is a small, thin segment of skin similar to a drum. The inner surface of the eardrum marks the beginning of the middle ear. The middle ear and inner ear are housed in the *temporal bone*, the hardest bone in the entire body.

Depending on their pitch and volume, sound waves have slightly different effects on the eardrum. The eardrum transforms sound waves into vibrations that are eventually transmitted to the brain. But thanks to clever design, the eardrum also has the ability to shut down access to the brain. This occurs when muscles in the middle ear—the *tensor tympani muscle* and the *stapedius muscle*—both tighten simultaneously, making the middle ear bones more rigid. The net effect is a muting of loud, low-pitched noises that could damage the inner ear.

Interestingly, this process is much more effective in birds than in humans, where it provides very little protection against noise-induced damage to the ears. But the muting effect gives us one significant advantage: It keeps the sound of our own voices from overwhelming our ears. It can also dampen noisy distractions in our surroundings so we can better hear the voices of those near us, a process sometimes referred to as the cocktail party effect. (In essence, the cocktail party effect refers to our ability to hear a single voice in situations involving multiple conversations and background noise. Although it most certainly involves the ears' ability to mute certain sounds, speech and language qualities play a role in the process as well.)

The *ossicles,* the three smallest bones in the body, are located on the inner side of the eardrum. Their individual names are hammer (*malleus*), anvil (*incus*), and stirrup (*stapes*). Through a series of motions, the ossicles relay vibrations from the eardrum to the *cochlea,* where they can be converted from mechanical energy to electrical energy via the tiny hair cells in the inner ear. Once sound vibrations are transformed into electrical energy, they can be shuttled to the brain.

A closer look at this process reveals that when sound waves hit the eardrum, the drum's taut surface vibrates. The vibration moves inward, where it first encounters the hammer, which is directly connected to the eardrum. The hammer then transmits the vibration to the next bone, the anvil, and that bone relays the movement to the stirrup. These three bones make up the *ossicular chain.* When vibrations reach the end of the chain, they cause changes in the base of the stirrup (technically known as *stapes footplate*), which is directly linked to the *oval window,* the beginning of the inner ear.

Inside the Inner Ear

The best-known part of the inner ear is undoubtedly the cochlea, made famous by cochlear implants, sophisticated devices that can be implanted in the ear to counteract hearing loss. The cochlea is a snail-shell-shaped bony tube that is flexible on the inside (cochlea actually means "snail shell" in Latin). Its function is to translate sound vibrations into nerve impulses. Since it is rolled up like a garden hose inside the inner ear, the cochlea packs a great deal into a very small space, no larger than a dime. The base of the cochlea responds to high-frequency sounds, whereas its apex reacts to low-frequency sounds.

The cochlea is a remarkable device, filled with two different fluids (*perilymph* and *endolymph*), extraordinarily delicate hair cells, and microscopic fibers. In addition, the cochlea houses the *organ of Corti*, named for Italian anatomist Alfonso Corti, who first identified it in 1850. The cochlea's highly sensitive hair cells are situated in the organ of Corti. There are four rows of hair cells—three outer rows and one inner row, for a grand total of approximately twenty thousand cells. Their primary function is to respond to pressure variations in the fluid-filled cochlea, and that information is sent, in the form of electrical impulses, to the brain's cerebral cortex via the *acoustic,* or *auditory, nerve.*

The hair cells fall into two different categories—outer hair cells and inner hair cells—and each type has a specific job. The outer hair cells are able to "turn up the volume" for the brain by amplifying sounds, as well as fine-tuning them. The inner hair cells serve primarily as messengers, sending signals to the brain for decoding. All these elements work together to process the sounds around us into information that can be interpreted by the brain.

HISTORY AND MYSTERIES OF HEARING

Physicist Georg von Bekesy won a Nobel Prize in 1961 for deciphering the inner workings of the ear and its various elements. However, there are still many unanswered questions about hearing that researchers are investigating. And new discoveries are fairly common. For example, British scientists recently found that the tiny outer hair cells in the inner ear actually make noise themselves. Ever on the alert for sounds in our surroundings, these bundles vibrate continuously. The resulting sound, which cannot be heard by the human ear, can be used to determine if newborn babies' hearing is functional. The technical name for these sounds is *otoacoustic emissions*.[1]

Hair Cells: The Keys to Hearing

Although all the elements making up the ear are important, the tiny hair cells are especially vital to good hearing. It is these cells that are damaged with age, noise, certain drugs, including some antibiotics, circulatory problems, genetics, diseases such as mumps, and infections.

Even though they are too small to be seen with the naked eye, the cochlea's hair cells play a vital role in helping the brain identify specific sounds, because certain hair cells respond to particular sounds. Imagine for a moment that we have built a larger-than-life working model of the cochlea. Uncoiled, it looks much like a strip of Velcro. Now if we submerge it in a bowl of water, to represent the cochlear fluid, the hair cells look like tendrils of seaweed floating in the water. If the doorbell rings, the only tendrils that will react are those that respond to the particular frequency of the doorbell's sound waves. Similarly, if someone were to begin practicing a cello, each note that was played would activate different tendrils. In other words, the hair cell activity provides the brain with very detailed information about the precise nature of the sound waves entering our ears.

The information collected and processed by the ears still needs to pass through the auditory nerves on both sides of the head to reach the brain. The data collected by both ears is relayed to both sides of the brain's *auditory cortex,* where there are a number of areas devoted to auditory input. Here, the auditory cortex synthesizes the sounds and allows us to interpret/understand what we are hearing. Since the inner workings of the brain are highly complex, and not completely understood, we can stop this portion of our tour here and take a look at another completely different aspect of the ear—the *vestibular system*—which has less to do with hearing and everything to do with our ability to walk upright.

Balance Begins in the Ears

The ears are more than command central for hearing. The inner ear houses the vestibular system, the name given to five organs that play an essential role in our ability to stand steadily in an upright position, as well as maintain equilibrium while performing complex tasks and movements. The vestibular system consists of three *semicircular canals,* the *utricle,* and the *saccule.*

Each of the semicircular canals, which resemble three tiny loops positioned near the cochlea, monitors a different type of movement by the head. The canals are something like partially filled bowls. When the body moves, the liquid (the same endolymph that fills the cochlea) in the semicircular canals moves, too. One canal reacts to horizontal movement, one to vertical, and one to the head tipping from one side to the other. The canals are equipped with tiny sensory hair cells that respond to the fluid's movement by relaying nerve impulses through the acoustic nerve to the brain. Drinking too much alcohol can lead to problems with the vestibular system, such as stumbling, weaving, and the head-spinning sensation that the room is revolving. Certain health conditions, such as Ménière's disease, can affect the inner ear's balance mechanisms, too.

Of course, you don't have to be intoxicated or ill to experience disruptions in your sense of balance. If you have ever found the world spinning after getting off a merry-go-round or other amusement park ride, it's because the ride disturbed the balance of fluids in the inner ears' semicircular canals. As noted above, when the body moves, the liquid in the semicircular canals moves, too. In fact, this is how the body senses acceleration or motion. But when the body stops moving, it takes a little longer for the fluid in the canals to settle down. During this transition period, the brain has to deal with conflicting messages—the body is moving normally, but the fluid in the semicircular canal is still going. As a result, you may feel woozy or dizzy until the fluid returns to normal.

The semicircular canals are devoted to monitoring the head's movement. Meanwhile, the other two elements in the vestibular system—the utricle and saccule—focus on the head when it is not moving. Like the semicircular canals, these two tiny organs contain sensory hair cells that send nerve impulses to the brain via the acoustic nerve.

The Physics of Hearing

Throughout these processes, complex reactions are occurring that involve sound waves, air pressure, fluid movement, and the science of physics. In this realm, the technical information can become quite daunting, but a little more detail will help make sense of some common occurrences related to the ears.

Why, for example, do we often have trouble hearing well when we have a cold? This is because the ears are connected to the outside world not just through the ear canal, but via the *Eustachian tube* as well. The Eustachian tube is a narrow tube that connects the middle ear to the back of the nose. And here we need a quick physics lesson. As we have seen, the eardrum is held taut. The eardrum's position relative to the middle ear is maintained by keeping the air pressure stable on both sides. When we have a head cold and our sinuses are inflamed and filled with mucus, the air pressure can't be equalized as efficiently, resulting in the "stuffy" or muffled feeling that blocks sound waves and makes hearing difficult.

This is the same mechanism that causes ears to "pop" during even a slight change in altitude, such as driving up or down a hill. That popping is simply the Eustachian tube opening to help maintain equal air pressure on both sides of the eardrum. Another common example occurs on an airplane, when the cabin is pressurized. This forces the eardrum to be pushed inward. Some people can open their Eustachian tubes by moving the jaw, chewing gum, swallowing, or yawning. For others, more force may be required, such as pinching the nose, closing the mouth, and gently blowing, a trick used by scuba divers to prevent ruptures of the eardrum or more serious damage.

Ear infections, one of the most common afflictions among babies and young children, are due to the fact that the Eustachian tubes are not fully developed until sometime between four and six years of age. The undeveloped tubes don't function properly, making children vulnerable to ear infections. This is why surgically inserting temporary "tubes" (also known as pressure-equalizing tubes or ventilation tubes) helps reduce recurring ear infections. The temporary tubes bypass a child's underdeveloped Eustachian tubes and allow the pressure to equalize. The tubes have been very successful at minimizing the misery of children's ear infections—not to mention parents' lost sleep—and this is now one of the most commonly performed surgical procedures.

Sources of Sounds

In order for our ears to do their job, of course, there must be something to hear. The sounds that reach our ears come from a variety of sources—voices, movement, musical instruments, mechanical equipment, and various devices—yet they are all basically the same. As we saw a little earlier in this chapter, sound is created by vibrations called sound waves.

> ### THE SCIENCE OF SOUND
>
> Air is essential for the transmission of sound. In its simplest terms, music is nothing more than air vibrations created with various materials and under different circumstances. There is no sound in outer space, however, because there is no air and therefore no sound waves. Communication must take place via radio waves, which are different than sound waves and can be transmitted in a vacuum.

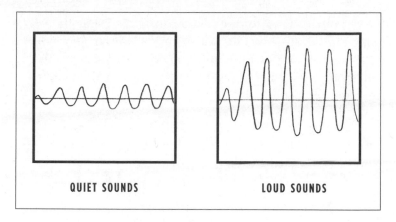

QUIET SOUNDS   **LOUD SOUNDS**

Figure 2: **Amplitude**

There are a wide range of sounds, including loud, soft, high, low, and some that we humans simply cannot hear. All these different sound waves have one thing in common: They travel at the same speed. The thing that makes one sound different from another is the shape of the sound wave. *Amplitude* determines whether a sound is loud or quiet. Loud sounds have high amplitude, meaning the sound waves create dramatic highs and lows in air pressure as they travel. Low-amplitude sounds produce less "wavy" sound waves, without the roller-coaster peaks and valleys of louder sounds.

Frequency is the aspect that determines whether a sound has a high or low pitch. When high-pitched sounds are compared to those with a low pitch, they create more vibrations during a one-second period. Therefore, high-frequency sound waves are high in pitch, while low-frequency waves are at the other end of the scale. For example, a flute produces high-frequency sounds, while drums are in the low-frequency range.

A sound wave's vibration is measured in a unit known as

a *hertz* (Hz), named for the German physicist Heinrich Hertz, who first identified radio waves in the nineteenth century. One hertz indicates one vibration in a second; megahertz (MHz) means 1 million hertz, the equivalent of 1 million vibrations per second.

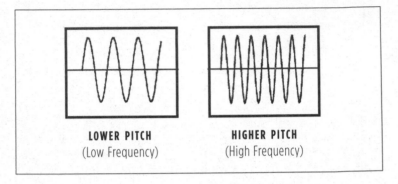

LOWER PITCH   **HIGHER PITCH**
(Low Frequency)   (High Frequency)

Figure 3: **Frequency**

LET'S HEAR IT FOR ANIMALS

Many animals and other creatures have a far better ability to hear than humans. Dogs, for example, register sounds as high as 50,000 Hz, while a bat's incredibly sensitive ears detect ultrasounds in the 120,000 Hz range. In humans, the ability to hear is best during the early years, when a child with normal hearing can sense sounds up to 20,000 Hz. During the teen years, that figure drops to 12,000 Hz. Somewhere between ages thirty-five and forty, we don't really hear very well if sounds are more than 9,000 to 10,000 Hz. After age fifty, that figure can fall to 4,000 to 8,000 Hz.

A *decibel* (dB) is a number commonly used to represent an intensity, strength, or power. Strength of a sound is roughly equivalent to its loudness, but is not technically the same thing. Named for Alexander Graham Bell, best known for inventing the telephone, the decibel scale is logarithmic. This means that an increase of ten dB—say from 10 dB to 20 dB, for example—is not twice as powerful, but *ten times* as strong! In other words, 10 is not added to the base number, but multiplied times it. So while a whisper usually falls in the 20 dB range, the sound of a hushed conversation at 30 dB is actually ten times louder than the whisper. (See table on page 3.)

As a general rule, we should avoid or minimize exposure to sounds in and above the 85 to 90 dB range. Higher levels, like 120 dB, can cause physical pain and damage hearing to the point of deafness. However, it's important to understand that the measure of a sound's intensity is not the only factor involved in noise-related hearing loss. There are two other aspects of sound to consider when assessing whether or not a noise is dangerous—frequency and time, or duration of exposure. An easy way to remember this is with the acronym FIT (Frequency, Intensity, and Time).

Frequency is roughly equivalent (but not identical) to pitch. Just as sound intensity is expressed in dB, frequency is expressed in Hertz (Hz) or cycles per second. Thus the high notes of a piano generate high frequencies and the ear treats that as a high pitch. The frequencies that cause the most damage to the ear are high frequencies up near the top of the piano (roughly 2,000 to 6,000 Hz).

Time is simply how long the ears are exposed to the sound. Obviously, a short session listening to a rock band or jackhammer will do far less harm to hearing than hours of exposure day after day, week after week.

Being aware of the FIT factors is critical to protecting hearing. Simply increasing the distance between your ears and the source of a sound, and decreasing the amount of time you can hear it reduces the risk of hearing loss. Understand, too, that the two types of hair cells are affected differently by the FIT factors. First of all, the inner hair cells need the help of the outer hair cells. The outer hair cells are amplifiers which respond to faint sounds, so when they are compromised two things happen: The cochlea fails to amplify faint sounds up to about 65 dB and a process known as "recruitment" occurs. Recruitment basically means that faint sounds, usually amplified by the outer cells, are not heard at all, but abruptly become audible when the sounds exceed roughly 65 dB. The inner hair cells can then respond normally to this more powerful sound just as effectively as if the outer hair cells were working. This leaves the listener with a very uneven sense of hearing connected speech. Some parts of a word are clear while other parts (those which fall below 65 dB) are inaudible. Similarly, when the inner hair cells are compromised, areas of the cochlea become non-functional "dead zones," a situation that cannot be corrected with hearing aids. Fortunately, the antioxidants and other nutrients in the Save Your Hearing Now Program are able to protect both the outer and inner hair cells and their mitochondria.

If all this information seems overwhelming, don't worry. Essentially, what you need to know is that the ear can be divided into three portions: outer ear (the part we can see), middle ear (site of the eardrum and hammer, anvil, and stirrup), and inner ear (where the cochlea's hair cells reside). Simply put, the basic process of hearing consists of sound vibrations entering the ear and being funneled through the ear canal to the eardrum. The vibrations then pass through the eardrum and move to the fluid-filled cochlea, where they create motion among the tens of thousands of hair cells. The hair cells then generate electrical impulses which are sent to the brain's auditory cortex for translation.

Now that you know how hearing works, let's take a look at how the changes that occur during aging, which are the leading causes of hearing loss, affects the auditory system, and get an idea of how the Save Your Hearing Now Program can prevent some of those changes from taking place.

((3))

HOW AGING AFFECTS HEARING AND WHAT WE CAN DO ABOUT IT

Three older gentlemen were making the rounds of the golf course one day. While waiting for a breeze to calm down, one said, "Windy, isn't it?"

"No," replied the second. "It's Thursday."

"So am I," agreed the third one. "How about a beer?"

Age-related hearing loss affects approximately one-third of all people aged sixty-five and older. Technically known as *presbyacusia* or *presbycusis,* age-related hearing loss is due to the changes that occur in the body as we grow older. Circulatory disorders, for example, which limit the flow of blood throughout the body, as well as to the brain and auditory system, are common in later years. There are any number of reasons why circulation slows down as we grow older, among them heart disease, hardening of the arteries, diabetes, and sedentary lifestyles. Oftentimes, however, lifestyle changes can postpone or overcome many of the medical conditions we commonly associate with advanced years.

Can science help us avoid or delay the often dire consequences of aging, including hearing loss? I say absolutely, and I am not alone. All over the world, scientists are working hard on developing ways to increase both the quality and the quantity of the years of the average human life. So far, there are promising signs that the aging process can be delayed. There are also encouraging results from our experimental work that the process can be halted, but it would be premature to say this applies to humans.

My research and that of many colleagues clearly show that the same things that protect us from the damage done by passing years also prevent damage to our hearing. In order to understand how hearing can be saved by slowing the clock, let's take a look at the aging process and what happens in the body, especially the auditory system, as time passes.

Aging Begins in the Cells

Without a doubt, longevity and antiaging research are hot topics in science these days. Obviously, a drug that could keep people young would be a huge best-seller. In order to develop an antiaging medication, however, scientists have to understand how aging works. Yet, in spite of years of research, there is no final answer to the question of why we grow old.

We do know a few things, though. During a normal lifetime, our cells divide anywhere from twenty to thirty times. This ongoing process of cellular expansion turns a child into an adult, and then cell division slows. Ultimately, because of inherent limits, our cells are no longer able to divide. (The *Hayflick limit,* named for Leonard Hayflick, the scientist who discovered it in 1961, is the term used to describe the number of times cell division can take place.) So although we continue to need new cells, later in life our bodies are not as efficient as they once were at producing them. The result: Disease or malfunctions occur because faulty cells are not replaced with fully functional versions.

In addition to the inherent limitations on new cell production, other factors are thought to play a role in aging. There are several different theories about the process, including the free-radical or mitochondrial clock theory, dysdifferentiation theory, and the telomerase theory. Thus far, the free-radical theory has the widest acceptance. Scientists also have a good idea of how it works and what we can do about it.

The Enemy: Free Radicals

In simplest terms, a *free radical* is an unstable molecule or cluster of molecules that is missing an electron. Like mini–atomic bombs, free radicals damage or destroy cells they come in contact with. Free radicals are by-products of everything from eating to living in a world filled with toxic chemicals and pollution. In other words, they are unavoidable. Although some free radicals are actually beneficial, others damage healthy cells. Free radicals can cause errors in genetic "messages" by altering DNA (deoxyribonucleic acid, the "blueprint" that governs cell growth). This can, among other things, lead to a reduced blood supply to organs such as the inner ear and brain, thereby damaging hearing.

When one of these loose cannon free-radical molecules binds with a healthy cell, it wreaks havoc on the cell's ability to function. Mother Nature did not leave us completely defenseless, though. Our bodies produce enzymes known as *antioxidants*—such as superoxide dismutase (SOD), catalase, and glutathione peroxidase—to counteract the damage. We can also obtain antioxidants from certain foods and supplements. But if inadequate production or a poor diet results in a shortage of antioxidants, cellular damage may not be repaired, and sooner or later, we become ill. There have been many studies documenting that free radicals are responsible for more than a hundred human diseases, including Alzheimer's, cancer, heart attacks, strokes, and arthritis, as well as aging.

Even though free radicals are microscopic and exist for far less time than it takes to blink an eye, they are capable of doing considerable damage simply because of their sheer numbers. According to research at Emory University, each human cell receives approximately ten thousand free-radical hits each day. Further calculations have shown that this equals 7 trillion (7,000,000,000,000!) insults per second throughout our bodies.[1]

Certainly, 7 trillion is a staggering number, but the body counteracts this assault with its own arsenal of antioxidant enzymes. Unfortunately, there is a significant decline in these enzymes as we grow older. In fact, we now know that by the time the average person reaches the late twenties, production of these detoxifying enzymes has declined dramatically. Based on the findings of scientists studying free radicals and human health, the best approach to slowing aging is one that provides the body with plenty of antioxidant ammunition against free radicals. That means increasing intake of antioxidants, something that can be done in part with the proper diet or, more effectively, by taking supplements.

The Mighty Mitochondria

To measure free-radical damage, scientists can look for certain "markers," chemical or cellular signposts that indicate change within a cell. In humans, one of these markers is known as the *common aging deletion*. It is a sign of both advancing years and free-radical damage to the DNA of tiny organelles within each cell known as *mitochondria*.

About 98 percent of our body's energy is produced in mitochondria, so they are often described as the cells' powerhouses. A number of studies have shown that the functions of the mitochondria decrease with age, leading some experts to speculate that this may be why many people feel less energetic as they grow older. The hardworking mitochondria also serve as the cells' "gatekeepers," with the power to determine whether a cell lives or dies, so it's doubly important to keep the mitochondria healthy.[2]

The mitochondria have their own DNA, which is completely separate from the DNA found in the cells. When free radicals ravage the cellular DNA, it can be repaired, but the mitochondria's cannot. The mitochondria can be weakened or may even die, creating a slowdown in many essential processes.

Even an incredibly small mutation in the mitochondrial DNA can dramatically slow energy production. In fact, the drop in mitochondrial activity is the basis of the free radical or mitochondrial clock theory of aging. According to this theory, the aging body increases its production of free radicals, which damage the body's tissues and subcellular elements, such as the mitochondria. When we see the common aging deletion in mitochondria, we know the cells' little energy factories aren't fully functioning.

Unraveling the Hearing Loss Mystery in the Lab

After treating hundreds of patients suffering from hearing loss—and seeing the devastating effects it had on their lives—I decided to look for a natural solution. Knowing that antioxidants counteract the damage caused by free radicals, I thought there might be a way to use those same safe, natural substances to protect and/or restore hearing. But first the fact that there was a link between free-radical damage and hearing loss had to be established. So the first study my colleagues and I conducted was designed to find out if there was a connection between damaged hearing in humans and the common aging deletion. (Little did I know that the search would also uncover several potent age-fighters, something we'll look at a little later.)

From previous research in our lab and by others, we knew four things:

1. Common aging deletions accumulate as we grow older.
2. Blood flow to the cochlea, home to the nerve endings that make hearing possible, decreases as we age.[3]
3. At the same time, our hearing apparatus becomes less sensitive.[4]
4. As we age, our bodies produce more free radicals and fewer of the antioxidants that protect our hearing from free-radical damage.[5]

To test the theory that aging damages hearing and common aging deletions are a sign of that damage, we examined the temporal bones (those found at the sides and base of the skull) of thirty-four individuals, seventeen with normal hearing and seventeen who had age-related hearing loss. Temporal bones, as we saw in Chapter Two, house the cochlea, the snail-shell-shaped organ responsible for hearing, and this is why we focused on that particular area. We found the common aging deletion in fourteen of the seventeen individuals with hearing loss and in eight of those with normal hearing.

Why didn't the deletion appear in all seventeen of those with hearing loss? And why did it appear in bones of people whose hearing was fine? At least two reasons: The common aging deletion is only one type of deletion. It could be that other deletions contribute to hearing loss, too. In addition, there are four different types of age-related hearing loss. The common aging deletion may not be responsible for all four. At any rate, this study provided us with enough evidence to conclude that the common aging deletion is associated with aging and hearing loss.[6]

Supporting the First Findings

The link between aging and hearing loss was underscored by our next study. It involved a number of rats, which were divided into four age groups: young, mid-young, mid-old, and old. We tested the sensitivity of rats' hearing and examined their DNA for the common aging deletion, to determine if there was an association between the two. We found that, like humans, rats tend to have higher levels of the common aging deletion as they grow older, and they have an increased tendency to develop hearing loss as well.[7]

Now we had established that the aging process resulted in an increase in common aging deletions, which weakened the mitochondria and damaged hearing. But could the damage be slowed, prevented, or possibly even repaired with supplements of naturally occurring antioxidants? That's the question we set out to answer with two additional studies.

In one clinical trial, we followed animals from approximately several months old to the day they died. One group received a calorie-restricted diet, shown to reduce free-radical production, reduce mitochondrial damage, and to increase life span. For purposes of comparison, a placebo-controlled group was allowed to eat freely. Other groups were treated with antioxidants, including vitamins E and C, and the hormone melatonin. With this study, we demonstrated that free radicals and damage to the mitochondria that occurs with aging leads to presbycusis, the medical term given to age-related hearing loss. Furthermore, we were able to demonstrate that dietary moderation and specific nutrients reduce the progression of age-related hearing loss, and we concluded that it is likely that a combination therapy would provide a synergistic protective effect on presbycusis and possibly on aging as well.[8]

But even more dramatic results occurred in our next clinical trial. In this study, we used twenty-one two-year-old rats, senior citizens in the rodent world, and divided them into three groups of seven each. For six weeks, one group was given ALC (acetyl-L-carnitine), the second was given ALA (alpha-lipoic acid), and the third group, used as a control, received a placebo (sugar pill).

If you're at all familiar with antioxidants, you know that there are quite a few out there, including some superstars. Why did we choose these lesser-known substances? Because both are widely researched and have demonstrated potent antiaging properties.

When we tallied the results, it was clear that hearing in the control (placebo) group had deteriorated at a rate typical for animals of that age. But that didn't happen with either group of supplemented animals. Instead, we discovered the ALA and ALC did something pretty amazing. The supplemented rats not only avoided hearing loss, but their hearing *actually improved*. In other words, supplements didn't just stop age-related hearing loss—they reversed it![9]

During the the study, the control group lost anywhere from 3 to 7 dB of hearing, while the ones treated with ALC or ALA had a 7 to 10 dB improvement in their hearing, with the greatest improvements occurring after six months of treatment. While the ALA was more effective for protecting hearing at low frequencies, ALC did better at higher frequencies. We demonstrated that taking *both* supplements is the best way to protect against hearing damage in general. This groundbreaking work was so novel that I was awarded a patent for this supplement.

Of all the research I've done, I consider this study the most important. It clearly demonstrates that hearing loss can be prevented—and even reversed—by simply taking a combination of antioxidants that includes ALA and ALC. Both these substances have been popular in Europe for some time, and are widely considered nontoxic, very effective in treating hearing loss, and also capable of providing overall antiaging and wellness benefits. And they are widely available in the United States at health food stores and vitamin shops. But there is another reason this study stands out. Medical research is full of surprises. Sometimes what makes perfect sense on paper just doesn't work in the lab. Other times we are literally astonished by the unanticipated benefits. That's what happened in this particular study. Along with improved hearing in the supplemented animals, we found a much lower level of common aging deletions in the mitochondria all throughout the body. That's right: The supplements actually reduced the amount of free-radical damage everywhere, creating an antiaging effect that improved hearing and carried over to other cells throughout the body—pretty exciting stuff! In other words, we had proven that age-related hearing loss can be reversed in mammals, with all-natural, side-effect-free substances. Although this research was groundbreaking at the time, other scientists have since shown that ALA, ALC, and various other substances, including the antioxidant coenzyme Q10 (coQ10) and glutathione, provide substantial protection for the mitochondria and thereby support healthy hearing.

TREATING AGE-RELATED HEARING LOSS WITH SUPPLEMENTS

"I know I'm not a kid anymore," Don told me, "but I'm in pretty good shape except for my hearing." Don was right on all counts. In his mid-sixties, he was trim, reasonably active, and well on his way to going deaf. Often, older individuals resign themselves to hearing loss and do nothing about it. But Don's thriving advertising consulting business was in jeopardy because he was having trouble understanding what his clients said on the telephone and in crowded meeting rooms. "As long as I have written instructions, everything's okay," he explained. "But I can't always get those."

To make matters worse, many of Don's clients were much younger than he was, so he felt that a hearing aid—even a small, discreet model—would make him look like an old-timer, to use his own words.

We discussed his lifestyle and found a number of places to make improvements. First, I encouraged him to wear hearing protection when he worked on his woodworking hobby, since he was using ear-damaging power tools. He agreed to eliminate some of the less healthful food choices from his diet and had no problem with increasing the time he spent exercising. But when it came to supplements, Don balked. "My doctor told me vitamins are a waste of money," he said firmly.

I explained that there is actually quite a large body of research showing that vitamins are beneficial and detailed some of my own research involving improved hearing. "You've already got so much going for you," I told him, "why not try supplements for a few months and see how it goes?"

Don said he would think about it and left. A few weeks later, he called and asked which supplements he should be taking. It turned out that he had misunderstood a client's directions for a project he was completing and been replaced by a younger competitor. Once the sting of losing the job was over, Don decided that if supplements could help with his hearing loss, they were worth a try.

About nine months passed before I heard from Don again. He called because he wanted to let me know that he was beginning to hear the birds chirping outside his bedroom window in the mornings. The sounds were still faint, but Don was excited by the improvement. "That hasn't happened in a long while," he said with a laugh. "I just thought I should let you know that you were right about those supplements."

What This Means to Us Humans

No doubt some of you are still a bit skeptical about all this. Maybe you're thinking something like, "Great news for lab rats! But I find it hard to believe the same stuff is going to work for me. Why don't researchers do these studies with people?" Here's why:

Duplicating these studies with humans would take several generations and cost hundreds of millions of dollars. But there are several advantages to working with rats. First, rats' ears are very similar to humans', so it is not much of a stretch to assume that anything that improves a rat's hearing would work with people, too.

Second, rats and humans tend to age in a similar fashion— except that rats do it far more quickly—so they are ideal for studying antiaging strategies. In a period of roughly two years, which is the typical rat's life span, we can see the effects of supplements, medications, and other treatments. If we did the same tests with humans, it is quite possible the researcher wouldn't be around long enough to see the results of the study. (By the way, all the animals in our studies are treated humanely, in accordance with NIH guidelines and guidelines set up for the care of experimental animals. These agencies place very strict protocols that must be followed precisely, for the welfare of the subjects.)

The proof that the program works has been amply demonstrated for me by the success stories I've heard from hundreds of patients. After so many people described how their lives changed—especially those who were skeptical to begin with—it became quite clear that hearing loss can be halted and sometimes corrected through the use of appropriate nutrients and lifestyle changes. And hearing isn't the only thing that is affected. A large number of patients report that their stress and anxiety levels plummeted once they discovered that they didn't have to worry about suffering further hearing loss or becoming completely deaf. Economically, this approach has helped many people, too. "Now I feel like I have more time to save up for a hearing aid," one older patient told me. "And I'm even keeping my fingers crossed that I won't need one!"

As I share more of these individuals' stories and triumphs and explain in greater detail how the program works, it will become clear that the bottom line is this: Save Your Hearing Now is nothing less than a simple, safe, and entirely revolutionary method of preventing hearing loss and, in some cases, even reversing hearing loss. Better hearing means better quality of life, and this program has been developed to provide just that.

The Lifestyle Connection

In addition to providing the body with adequate amounts of antioxidants and other important nutrients, we've also discovered that there are several other things we can do to slow aging and save hearing. One good place to begin is by accepting responsibility for your health, and not succumbing to the idea that genes rule. Certainly, our parents and older siblings can give us some indication of what might lie ahead. But biology is not necessarily destiny. Several studies have shown that a healthy lifestyle trumps genetics.

Here is a great example: In a study involving sets of healthy twins, researchers in Finland kept track of the twins' lifestyles for nearly twenty years. At the end of the study, they discovered that those who exercised moderately—thirty minutes of walking twice a week—cut their risk of dying almost in half when compared to their sedentary sibling.[10]

Individual differences have a profound effect on the aging process. Right now it is impossible to predict how the passage of time will change a person. But research is showing the tremendous importance of lifestyle to the aging process. To illustrate, let's compare two fifty-year-old individuals. One person lives at sea level, is an appropriate weight, eats a healthful diet consisting of significant amounts of fruits and vegetables, limits alcohol consumption, exercises regularly, and practices stress management techniques. The second person lives in Aspen, Colorado, at 7,800 feet above sea level, where he is exposed to more ionizing radiation from the sun than a person living at lower altitude. In addition, he is fifty pounds overweight, eats fast food daily, smokes and drinks excessively, considers stress to be a myth, and does not exercise.

Although both of these individuals are chronologically fifty years old, molecularly they are quite different. In fact, mitochondrial DNA analysis would show that the fifty-year-old living in Aspen has DNA damage that would be associated with an approximately seventy-year-old human. This means that the cells throughout his body, including those in the auditory system, are not able to function at optimal levels. It would not be at all surprising to find chronic age-related health problems, such as osteoarthritis, cognitive difficulties, and, of course, hearing loss in this individual.

Meanwhile, the fifty-year-old living at sea level with a very healthy lifestyle has the DNA damage of a thirty-year-old. His cells are able to perform all their functions, so his auditory system and all other organs are likely to be in top working order.

As this example shows, lifestyle is closely linked to how we age, with eating habits and activity taking the lead roles.

Living on Less: The Lowdown on Caloric Restriction

A major aspect of the lifestyle-aging connection is the food an individual chooses to eat. Good food can provide us with ample supplies of antioxidants, while less nutritious fare can stimulate production of damaging free radicals. There is very thorough documentation, for example, that certain foods— such as fatty and processed meats—lead to a significant increase in free-radical production.

Eating high-quality food clearly supports good health at the cellular level. But science has taken that approach one step further. Research going back more than seventy years shows that "caloric restriction," the term given to low-calorie, high-nutrient diets, extends the life span of laboratory animals and insects by up to 50 percent. In fact, nearly two thousand studies have confirmed the connection between caloric restriction and extended life span in a number of different species.

Of course, here again, it is not practical or feasible to have human beings as test subjects in longevity experiments. Instead, test subjects that have well-documented life expectancies are used. The average protozoa on a normal diet, for example, are typically alive for seven to fourteen days. On a caloric-restriction program, though, the average protozoan life span is thirteen days and can go as long as twenty-five, nearly double the maximum with a standard diet.

Caloric restriction is currently a hot topic among scientists studying longevity, primarily because it works so well. What does a restricted-calorie diet look like? Most of us would not find it a pretty sight. Based on what we know now, to achieve life extension results, we would have to eliminate 30 percent or more of our daily calorie intake. According to the Calorie Restriction Society (http://www.cron-web.org), four daily meals should add up to no more than 1,700 to 1,800 calories. Most people are simply not willing to trade away so many calories for additional years.

It probably wouldn't hurt most of us to cut back a little at mealtime, though. And it is possible that hearing could improve as a result, because caloric restriction is shaping up as a means of protecting more than the waistline. The benefits of skipping extra calories appear to extend to the brain, where much of the auditory system is located. A recent animal study at the University of Wisconsin, Madison, reported in *Nature Genetics*, demonstrated that a reduced-calorie diet actually protects brain cells from deterioration caused by aging, the very types of changes that could lead to Alzheimer's and other degenerative conditions.[11] In fact, two other studies that examined patients with Parkinson's determined that high-calorie diets were linked to the likelihood of developing the disease.[12] So skip the dessert and do your waist—and your brain—a favor.

The good news is that you don't have to starve yourself to save your hearing. Choosing foods that are high in antioxidants is the key, and we will look at ways to do that in Chapter Seven.

Move It or Lose It

Food can protect against age-related hearing loss by keeping antioxidant levels high. Activity has a different role. When we are active—whether it's playing golf, riding a bike, or simply walking around the block—circulation is stimulated. Good circulation is vitally important to good overall health, as well as good hearing. A sedentary lifestyle does not provide adequate circulation throughout the body, so the auditory system is deprived of the oxygen, antioxidants, and other nutrients it needs. The cochlea, for example, requires a continually renewed blood supply to function properly, and the same is true for all of the body's organs.

In our lifestyle example, you may recall that the "younger" fifty-year-old was active and had no hearing loss, while the "older" one, who did not exercise, had difficulty hearing. Unfortunately, in our sedentary society, exercise is one of the most overlooked—or should I say avoided?—means of delaying aging. Study after study has shown that physical activity helps relieve many of the disorders commonly associated with aging—heart disease in particular. For example, new research from Albert Einstein College of Medicine demonstrated that individuals who exercised regularly had a lower risk of heart attack, and those with high blood pressure benefited most from physical activity.[13]

A healthy cardiovascular system is especially important to good hearing, because it plays a major role in circulation. It would be premature to say that the connection between a healthy heart and good hearing has been firmly established. But there are certainly strong indications that the two go hand in hand. Research presented at an American Heart Association meeting in 2002 showed that individuals with cardiovascular disease were nearly 55 percent more likely to have hearing loss related to cochlear malfunctions than people who did not have heart disease. The same study noted that individuals with a history of a heart attack are more likely to experience hearing difficulties because the cochlea is compromised.[14] Regular exercise is a fundamental element of the Save Your Hearing Now Program. More information on physical activity as it relates to hearing, as well as guidelines for creating your own personal exercise program, can be found in Chapter Nine.

How Drugs Damage Hearing

Making age-fighting lifestyle changes can benefit hearing in another, very significant way. It is a little-known fact that many commonly prescribed drugs are *ototoxic,* or damaging to hearing. There are hundreds of ototoxic drugs, including popular nonsteroidal anti-inflammatory drugs (NSAIDs), like aspirin, as well as some antidepressant and antianxiety drugs, to name a few. Typically, people taking these medications have no idea that their hearing could be affected. Moreover, since the hearing loss may not appear until months after beginning the medication, the connection is far from obvious. The medication is rarely suspected to be the source of the problem, and every prescription refill continues the hearing damage.

A younger person may have more resistance to drugs that damage hearing, and is more likely to be taking only one or two medications at a time. Increasingly, though, older people are prescribed multiple remedies for a host of ailments that occur later in life. Often, these medications are prescribed by different doctors, who may not be aware of the total number of medications the patient is taking. The compound effect of taking multiple drugs—and its impact on hearing—are completely unknown. But certainly, if an individual is taking more than one ototoxic medication—and one is all it takes to damage hearing—we can assume the results are not going to be good.

Drugs can be lifesavers, to be sure. But in addition to hearing loss, there are other downsides. For example, each year, approximately 100,000 people in this country are hospitalized for health problems related to pharmaceutical drugs. According to a survey from the American Association of Retired Persons (AARP), many of these cases are caused by a "medication information gap."

Drug companies are increasingly advertising "prescription-only" products directly to consumers, in part to create public awareness of new remedies. But frequently, older individuals don't notice the ads' fine print, where information about a drug's side effects and risks are listed. In fact, the AARP survey found that less than half of those individuals aged sixty and older are aware of this essential information. A related problem stems from a lack of communication between patients and health care professionals. Only 54 percent of those polled by the AARP said their pharmacist or doctor "usually" discusses a drug's potential dangers with them. Clearly, this is an area where patients need to "take charge" of their own health by asking plenty of questions.

POPULAR DRUGS AND HEARING DAMAGE

Literally hundreds of drugs can affect the ability to hear, including popular nonsteroidal anti-inflammatory drugs (NSAIDs), like aspirin. In many cases, large doses or abuse of a drug can cause hearing loss, but when the same medication is taken as prescribed, it does not harm hearing. In normal doses, aspirin, for example, is considered safe, but those individuals who believe that "more is better" may be risking their hearing. One dramatic example occurred not long ago when talk show host Rush Limbaugh became deaf, an event that was eventually linked to his overdose of the prescription painkiller Vicodin. Other commonly prescribed drugs that affect hearing are:

- Antibiotics, including those classified as aminoglycosides (gentamicin, streptomycin, neomycin), macrolides (erythromycin, azithromycin), and vancomycin
- Loop diuretics (also known as furosemide or Lasix), which reduce the amount of fluid accumulating in the tissues
- Chemotherapeutic agents (oxaliplatin, cisplatin, carboplatin) used to treat various types of cancer
- Quinine-based antimalarial drugs
- Salicylate analgesics (large doses of aspirin)
- The pain reliever naproxen sodium (Naprosyn, Aleve), ibuprofen, and many other NSAIDs
- Some antidepressant and antianxiety medications

Keep in mind that hearing loss is not the only effect these substances may have on the auditory system. Tinnitus and problems with balance may also occur. In fact, individuals with tinnitus should be certain their physician is aware of their condition and request prescriptions that will not make the condition worse.

Drug-related hearing loss, as well as tinnitus and balance problems, may be temporary or permanent, depending on a number of factors, such as dosage and length of time the drug is taken.

Another method of reducing the likelihood of drug-related hearing loss is by making some simple alterations in lifestyle. In other words, if you improve your health, you need fewer drugs. Good nutrition and moderate physical activity have repeatedly been shown to improve symptoms in a host of conditions that are typically treated with pharmaceuticals, including depression, anxiety, arthritis, heart disease, diabetes, and high blood pressure. Some people find that making lifestyle changes allows them to use less medication, while others are able to work with their physician to gradually eliminate drugs completely. Either way, hearing and overall health benefit. For more information on drugs and hearing loss, see page 62.

"Old age is not for sissies," someone once said, and few people would argue. Many middle-aged people see their own parents' declining health, which usually includes some level of hearing loss, and are understandably concerned. But it's important to remember that today we know far more than ever before about the effects that the aging process has on hearing. Much of that knowledge involves nutrients and behavior that can slow—and possibly halt or even reverse—the cellular changes associated with age-related hearing damage. Many experts agree that next to the fountain of youth, the combination of nutritious eating, proper supplementation, and regular physical activity is the most potent antidote to hearing loss. Understand, though, that you don't have to be older or even experiencing hearing difficulties for the program to work. The same steps can be equally effective as preventative measures to maintain good hearing. And that is why these three elements (plus hearing protection) are cornerstones of the Save Your Hearing Now Program.

((4))

NOISE AND OTHER HEARING DAMAGE CULPRITS

There is no doubt that aging is the primary cause of hearing loss. But these days, noise is easily in second place. Not that long ago, many of the sounds we now take for granted—traffic, for instance, or telephones, appliances, and the ubiquitous sound systems broadcasting music in public places—simply did not exist. Individuals who grew up in quieter times—before World War II, for example—recall how unusual it was to hear a plane fly overhead or a car driving down a country road. Today, our lives are so filled with sound that it's very common to experience some level of hearing damage because of it and fairly challenging to find silence.

To get an idea of just how pervasive noise has become, let's spend a day with "Jackie," a typical adult who is completely unaware that the noise from her surroundings and everyday activities is slowly and steadily eroding her hearing.

A normal day for Jackie starts when her alarm clock buzzes her awake at 7:00 a.m. She gets up and takes a shower, using the exhaust fan to help eliminate moisture that steams up the bathroom mirror. Then Jackie uses the blow-dryer to fix her hair, gets dressed, and heads for the kitchen.

Like so many of us, Jackie enjoys a morning cup of freshly brewed coffee, which requires her to grind coffee beans and turn on the coffeemaker. At the same time, she whips up a smoothie in her blender and watches an early morning news show on TV while she waits for the honking horn signaling the arrival of her car pool.

In the car, Jackie and her co-workers simultaneously talk and listen to the radio, turning up the volume when a fire truck races by with its sirens blaring. They arrive at the office, where Jackie spends her day in a workstation, surrounded by her computer, a printer, fax machine, copier, four-line phone, and a PA system that is used for announcements about every half hour. For lunch, she walks to a fast-food restaurant with friends, then returns to her workstation for four more hours. After work, Jackie rides home with the car pool. The radio news competes with her co-workers' tales of the day's events.

At home, Jackie puts on a personal stereo headset and listens to some classical music while she goes for a quick jog. Afterward, she talks to her mother on her cell phone, runs the vacuum cleaner in the bedroom and living room, and showers before setting off to meet friends at a favorite restaurant, where a new trio is performing. Between the crowd in the restaurant and the musicians, it's hard for Jackie to hear herself think, let alone carry on a conversation. So after several hours of shouting and straining to hear, Jackie calls it a day and heads home. The long day has given her a headache, so before she turns in, Jackie takes a couple of aspirin and then turns out the light and goes to sleep.

Sound Measures

Let's take a closer look at the amount of noise generated by some of these examples, to see how Jackie's day is harming her hearing. The sound level from common appliances varies widely. An alarm clock, for example, can be fairly quiet, but if a heavy sleeper has to be awakened with either a screeching alarm or earsplitting music—typically in the 85 to 105 dB range—hearing suffers. Blow-dryers and bathroom exhaust fans, on the other hand, are fairly predictable in terms of noise. Blow-dryers can generate from 85 to 90 dB, while exhaust fans typically produce 90 dB or more.

The kitchen is a major source of modern-day noise. Jackie's coffee bean grinder probably creates 90 dB of sound, the blender 85 to 95 dB. Meanwhile, the combined drone of the coffeemaker (55 dB), refrigerator (50 dB), dishwasher (55 to 70 dB), and garbage disposal (80 to 95 dB) compounds the problem. Background noise from typical TV audio contributes another 70 dB.

As for the daily commute, the noise level can vary tremendously. Sounds associated with traveling in freeway traffic range from 70 to 85 dB. Throw in car pool companions plus a radio, and the noise level inside the car can easily hit the 90 dB range. The siren from the fire truck typically registers 150 dB, and automobile horns contribute about 110.

If Jackie uses public transportation, she's no better off. Using various means of transportation can also involve exposure to high levels of noise. A British audiologist measured sound on the London Underground and found levels reached as high as 188 dB, making them noisier than a jet engine or a jackhammer.[1] Surely, the average subway in the United States is just as loud as those in England, so for people who ride the trains on a regular basis, the accumulated damage of the daily commute could translate into permanent hearing loss.

Noise in the Workplace

Since Jackie has an office job, it might seem that her hearing is fairly safe during work hours. But today's workplace is typically filled with humming, whirring, buzzing, and ringing technology that is cumulatively responsible for 40 to 50 dB of ongoing background noise. And that's not counting the 80 dB of noise produced by a ringing telephone. Of course, the situation could be far worse. If Jackie worked in certain other industries—agriculture, manufacturing, construction, transportation, or as a musician, for example—her hearing could be in even more serious jeopardy.

Often, noise-induced hearing loss (NIHL) occurs on the job. The Occupational Safety and Health Administration (OSHA) has guidelines designed to protect individuals whose work places them at high risk for NIHL. (See page 234 in Resources.) But the guidelines are not always met.

One of the more difficult aspects of dealing with occupational noise is that people tend to become accustomed to it or consider it to be a simple fact of life. Oftentimes, too, individuals are concerned that complaining about noise levels or asking that something be done to minimize noise may not be appreciated by management or could put their job at risk. Even asking a co-worker to turn down her radio can create friction and resentment, so many people simply grin and bear it.

Another problem arises in job settings where noise-minimizing devices aren't appropriate. In the emergency room, for example, it's easy to see why—for doctors and nurses to work effectively, they cannot block the sound of voices and paging systems. Members of construction crews are frequently subjected to high levels of noise on the job, too, but again, eliminating noise means eliminating communication, so they live with the noise. Fortunately, technology can help deal with these problems. Today, there are ear protective devices available that screen out noise but allow voice frequencies to be heard. Too few people know about these, though, so those affected continue to be exposed to excessive noise.

No matter where you work or spend your day, here's the bottom line: The noise from everyday appliances, electronics, the environment, and occupation-related sounds, our lifestyles, and many commonplace drugs have a cumulative effect on our ability to hear. Experts at the National Institute on Deafness and Other Communication Disorders estimate that 10 million Americans have suffered irreversible hearing damage from noise, while another 30 million are exposed to dangerous noise levels each day, and these figures are considered conservative. Hearing loss is one of the top ten work-related health problems in the world, and the number of people in this category grows larger each day.

THE QUIET COMPUTER MOVEMENT

Computer noise may not seem like something to be concerned about, given other, much louder sources of environmental sound. But there is a small but growing number of people who are finding ways to reduce the continual low hum generated by computers, most of which comes from the movement of disk drives and cooling fans.

Computer-generated sound levels tend to be low in most machines. Those used for game-playing can register in 50 dB or more, but the average home or office computer usually reaches no more than 35 dB. Throughout Europe and parts of Scandinavia, however, where noise is more closely regulated by the government than in the United States, even these low levels of sound may be unacceptable. As a result, major computer manufacturers are developing quieter machines and marketing their low-noise features in the United States and abroad. Meanwhile, many individuals are creating custom modifications to minimize noise. For more information on the quiet computing movement and how to reduce computer noise, visit www.silent-pcreview.com or www.7volts.com.

More Noise in the Nighttime

When Jackie returns home in the evening, the noise level in her life remains high. Personal music devices—DiscMan, iPods, MP3 players, and the like—are tremendously popular. The problem is that many people crank up the volume to dangerously high levels. Set on high volume, these devices can generate 130 or more dB, more than the average rock concert! (As a rule of thumb, if you are wearing headphones to listen to music and a person standing next to you can hear the music, even faintly, the volume is too high.)

Cell phones are also hugely popular. In this case, though, we are dealing not only with the annoying, and sometimes overly loud, ring tones easily in the 70 dB range, but with unknowns in terms of the phones' effect on the body's cells and possible link to tumors, a highly controversial subject that is still open to debate.

When Jackie runs the vacuum cleaner, she is very likely being exposed to 85 to 90 dB of noise and there is another encounter with the exhaust fan in the bathroom during her evening shower. Needless to say, Jackie's evening out is not a hearing-friendly experience, either. The noise levels of restaurants vary widely, but add live music to the mix and it's easy for the decibel level to hit as much as 110 dB, depending on the sound system and how close Jackie is to the speakers.

Finally, let's look at the last item on the list—the aspirins Jackie takes at the end of the day. Considering all the favorable publicity and positive research results demonstrating aspirin's health benefits, many people are surprised to find this commonplace medication being mentioned as a threat to hearing. Here's the good news: Conservative doses of aspirin (for example, the daily 81 milligrams recommended for heart health) are not the problem. Many people, though, treat aspirin as a harmless remedy for whatever ails them—headache, hangover, muscle soreness, joint pain, you name it. People tend to pop aspirin without a second thought, and the steady intake over a period of time can affect hearing.

Of course, aspirin is not alone. An enormous number of popular drugs—especially prescription pharmaceuticals—can have very detrimental effects on hearing, as we saw earlier in Chapter Three.

The Link Between Our Noisy World and Hearing Loss

Needless to say, as the world becomes noisier, hearing loss increases. Between 1971 and 1990, according to the National Health Interview Survey, hearing problems among individuals between the ages of forty-five and sixty-four soared by 26 percent, and 17 percent of those queried in the eighteen to forty-four age group had hearing loss. We have to assume noise is primarily to blame, because none of these people are old enough to lose their hearing due to aging. Similarly, another survey, this one conducted in California and covering thirty years, found that middle-aged men (between the ages of fifty and fifty-nine) experienced a staggering 150 percent increase in hearing loss! There is even a new word to describe hearing loss that is not necessarily related to occupational noise: *sociocusis*!

BIG NOISE, LITTLE EARS

These days, even youngsters are being exposed to painfully loud sounds. Many parents believe that infants and small children are safe, since they're not in the iPod/cell phone age group. Not true! A large number of toys, including such things as musical "instruments," tricycle and bike horns, and "talking" electronic gadgets—all designed for very young children—make sounds that register in the 90 dB range or higher. Of course, anyone who has spent much time in a preschool environment or at a child's birthday party knows that children don't need any help when it comes to making noise. But screeching, beeping, wailing toys are a relatively new phenomenon, and one that parents should be aware of, because the whole family suffers.

A child's hearing can be damaged even before birth. It would seem that a fetus, safely ensconced in the womb, would be protected from loud noise by the fluids surrounding it, as well as by the mother's body. But several studies have shown hearing loss and other noise-related health issues (premature birth and decreased birth weight among them) in children who were born to women who spent time in noisy environments during pregnancy. [2]

Ironically, premature babies are often placed in the neonatal intensive-care unit (NICU), where again research has shown that noise-related hearing damage can occur, as well as a disruption of normal growth and development. Fortunately, when the noise in an NICU is reduced, these effects are eliminated. [3]

In many countries, pregnant women are prevented by law from working in environments where noise levels exceed certain standards. Those regulations are not always enforced, though, and they don't cover recreational or nonworking noise exposure, either. So a pregnant woman may attend an event like the symphony (80 dB or more) or a football game (110 dB in the stadium) not realizing that she could be harming her child's hearing. (If you would like more details on this very important issue, the American Academy of Pediatrics Committee on Environmental Health has issued a position paper titled "Noise: A Hazard for the Fetus and Newborn," which is available online at the following address: www.pediatrics.org/cgi/content/full/100/4/724.)

In spite of a considerable body of evidence linking noise

exposure with problems in childhood, few women—or men, for that matter—are aware of the effects noise can have on children. We have been warned for years that drinking is dangerous for pregnant women, and second-hand smoke has received tremendous publicity as a threat to children's health. But where are the warnings about noise exposure?

Not surprisingly, a recent study published in the journal *Pediatrics* reported noise-induced hearing loss in 12.5 percent of children between the ages of six and nineteen.[4] This figure may not seem exceptional, until you consider that not so long ago hearing loss was normally seen only in senior citizens well into their seventies or eighties. In other words, the noisy world we live in is taking a significant toll on hearing in all age groups.

The bottom line is that Americans—and baby boomers in particular—are losing their hearing almost twenty years earlier than the previous generation. What does this mean to our friend Jackie? If she is about thirty years old, it's very likely that in ten or fifteen years she will be at a party, in a busy restaurant, or at a meeting and realize that she is having trouble hearing conversations. Because hearing loss occurs so gradually, Jackie may unwittingly compensate for small changes over the years and deny anything is wrong. But one day, her hearing loss could reach the point at which it interferes with daily life. Then a situation that has been primarily frustrating, and at times embarrassing, can become life-threatening, as warnings, directions, or instructions are misunderstood.

The Noise Never Stops

There are plenty of examples and statistics showing how noisy the world has become, but let's just look at one more. In 1973, the Department of Housing and Urban Development (HUD) began the Annual Housing Survey, polling Americans on what they find dissatisfying about their neighborhoods. Without fail, noise is listed as a leading source of discontent each year, with close to 50 percent of the respondents naming noise as a major neighborhood problem. In addition, aircraft and traffic noise—not crime or gang violence—are the two primary reasons for moving from a neighborhood.[5]

When they look at the tremendous number of sounds and other factors in daily life that can diminish hearing, many people become frustrated and feel the situation is hopeless. Most of us cannot pack up and move easily, or quit a job simply because the workplace is a bit loud. The issue of hearing damage from drugs also causes a major dilemma for many individuals, who wonder if, to prevent damage to their hearing they have to endure arthritis pain or stop taking much-needed antidepressants.

Fortunately, I am not proposing anything quite so radical. Oftentimes, simply switching to a different medication eliminates the threat to hearing. And following the Save Your Hearing Now Program will provide a certain amount of protection from noise. To further reduce noise-related damage to hearing, however, it's important to be aware of the risk factors and avoid them whenever possible. Maybe you can't give up the blow-dryer, for example, but you might be able to live without the noisy luxury of freshly ground coffee beans. Or you may decide to continue all your normal activities but to wear earplugs or noise-reducing earmuffs at certain times, such as when mowing the lawn (95 dB) or while traveling on the subway (90 to 115 dB). In Chapter Nine, we'll take an in-depth look at earplugs and other protective devices.

NOISE POLLUTION HURTS EVERYONE

The notion that noise could be a pollutant first gained traction in the 1970s. The findings from more than three decades of studies examining the negative effects of noise on human health have shown how detrimental it can be, with potentially serious consequences far beyond damaged hearing. These include elevated stress, heart disease, high blood pressure, increases in the production of certain hormones to potentially damaging levels, and emotional distress. Adults aren't the only ones affected; numerous studies have shown that noise pollution harms the health and learning abilities of children, too.

Anyone who has had concentration or sleep interrupted by nearby construction, a late-night party, or a blasting car alarm knows how stressful noise can be, and researchers have repeatedly confirmed the link between noise and excessive stress. In addition, the physical effects noise has on us have been amply demonstrated. A number of studies, for example, have proven a strong connection between exposure to common noise sources, such as traffic, and high blood pressure.[6] And the damaging effects of noise on heart health was illustrated in a recent German study in which scientists found that both air and noise pollution heightened the risk of heart attacks. Yet while air pollution had negative effects on individuals who had a history of heart attacks, noise pollution caused an astonishing 140 percent increase in the likelihood of a heart attack in otherwise healthy individuals.[7]

Noise does not have to be steady or ongoing to be harmful to the heart. Consider, for example, the *startle response*, the body's reaction to a sudden, brief, usually loud noise. When a car backfires, for example, most people experience a startle response, usually characterized by blinking, jumping, or jerking, along with a little surge in adrenaline, the hormone that activates the body's fight-or-flight response. Not surprisingly, the first study to examine the health effects of the startle response found that substantial elevations in blood pressure and heart rate are involved in the process.[8]

High blood pressure and excessive levels of stress hormones were also found in children exposed to noise. But in addition, researchers noted that children in noisy environments also had problems with long-term memory and reading comprehension. Fortunately, when noise was removed from the children's environment, their symptoms subsided. In other words, eliminating noise restored their physical and emotional health.[9]

In addition to compromised physical health, noise has been shown to have psychological effects, such as reducing motivation among both children and adults. An Austrian study involving children found diminished motivation among young girls in noisy environments.[10] Recently, researchers examined the effects of low-level noise on women working in offices with open floor plans. When levels of stress hormones from the women in the moderately noisy setting were compared with those from women in quiet surroundings, there were significantly higher amounts of those potentially damaging hormones in the noisy group. Motivation was reduced as well. The women in noisier settings made 40 percent fewer attempts to solve a very difficult puzzle. Here again, the noisy environment was not particularly loud; researchers purposely wanted to test the effects of low-intensity office noise, not jet engine levels.[11]

If noise is a problem in your community, check out the Citizens Coalition Against Noise Pollution (NoiseOFF) at http://www.noiseoff.org. The organization provides dozens of articles and other information on all forms of noise pollution, including motorcycles, car alarms, neighbors, boom cars, and landscaping (leaf blowers and lawn mowers). In addition, NoiseOFF hosts an e-mail group where you may be able to find others in your area who are working to eliminate noise pollution, and/or get ideas on how to deal with the situation.

Another great source of information: the Noise Pollution Clearinghouse (NPC), a national nonprofit group with an enormous collection of online noise-related resources. Reducing noise in classrooms, on lakes, and on lawns and silencing car alarms are some areas NPC is focusing on. Visit www.nonoise.org for details.

Noise pollution receives very little public attention. The federal government awareness campaign, Wise Ears, sponsored by the National Institute on Deafness and Other Communication Disorders (see page 234 in Resources), is a worthwhile effort, but much more needs to be done to combat noise pollution. In addition, we should all make an effort to avoid noise whenever possible. When noise can't be escaped, we should use protective devices (practice "safe hearing," so to speak) and not be embarrassed by the fact that we consider our hearing to be worth saving.

A Closer Look at Hearing Loss

Technically speaking, there are three types of hearing loss: conductive, sensorineural, and central. In this book, we are primarily concerned with *sensorineural hearing loss* (SNHL). *Conductive hearing loss* is the name given to a condition that occurs when sound is not able to reach the inner ear. The stuffy feeling that comes with a bad head cold, ear infection, or allergies can cause temporary conductive hearing loss, because fluid in the ear interferes with transmission of sound.

Conductive hearing loss can also be caused by a perforated eardrum, excessive earwax, problems with the Eustachian tube, or deformities in the outer or middle ear, such as fixation of the middle ear bones. Whatever the cause, the result is that sounds are muffled and seem to be coming from far away, which is not the same as what occurs with SNHL. By and large, conductive hearing loss can be corrected. Colds, allergies, ear infections, and impacted earwax are treatable, and often, surgery can fix structural problems.

Central hearing loss, on the other hand, is a far more serious—and rare—condition. Generally, it involves brain damage, and it is not easily treatable.

Let's take a more in-depth look at SNHL. From a medical standpoint, there is little difference between the hearing damage that occurs at a rock concert and the changes that take place as we age. Minimizing noise exposure, therefore, is an excellent way to protect against hearing loss.

As we learned earlier, the cochlea of the inner ear contains thousands of tiny hair cells that transmit sounds to the brain. These hair cells are extraordinarily delicate, unable to withstand assaults from loud noises for very long. In addition, aging, many different drugs, birth or head trauma, an assortment of illnesses, genetic disorders, and tumors can be added to the list of SNHL causes, along with damage to the nerves that connect the inner ear and the brain.

Like conductive hearing loss, SNHL can cause sounds to seem muffled. But there is another hearing change that occurs with SNHL. While sounds at the low and mid-range of the spectrum come through clearly, high-frequencies do not register as efficiently. As a result, certain words are not clear. This is especially true if the speaker is a woman or a child, since their voices tend to fall in a higher-frequency range than men's. Consonants such as *P* and *T* can also be difficult to hear.

Generally, the first place most people with SNHL notice a problem is in a crowded or noisy setting, like a busy restaurant or a meeting room. "Bad acoustics" are often blamed, because in a quieter setting with less background noise, the problem is not nearly so noticeable. But once the cochlea's hair cells have been injured by repeated exposure to loud noises or age-related cellular changes, the damage has been done.

As you may recall from Chapter Two, specific hair cells in the cochlea are activated by certain sounds. When the cells are confronted with the same-frequency sound consistently, the hair cells' supportive structure becomes swollen and can rupture, destroying the hair cell. If enough hair cells in this region of the cochlea die, certain sounds may not be relayed to the brain, or the signal may be distorted, so that the brain interprets the sound incorrectly.

Let's say, for example, that the cluster of hair cells that recognize the middle C note is subjected to continuous, very loud repetitions of middle C. After a time, those cells die. The surrounding cells still relay information about music, but whenever middle C occurs, the brain does not receive the signal. In real life, this scenario is not likely to occur. In fact, very loud, high-decibel sounds that are also high in frequency, such as gunshots or factory equipment, are the most damaging, because they assault the ears with the maximum number of sound waves and the greatest force.

In some ways, the hair cells can be compared to a thriving, healthy lawn. The grass can accommodate a certain amount of wear and tear without being noticeably changed. But if certain areas are constantly trampled, the grass becomes worn down and eventually may die out in the sections where the hardest use occurs.

Fortunately, our hair cells are remarkably forgiving. If you have ever been to a rock concert or other extremely loud event, you may have had difficulty hearing clearly for a day or two afterward. Your ears may have felt like they had cotton in them, and you may have heard ringing or buzzing.

This condition is known as *temporary threshold shift* (TTS) and suggests significant trauma to the inner ear and cochlea. Repeated episodes of TTS, however, can eventually result in *permanent threshold shift* (PTS) and considerable hearing loss. For this reason, it's important to protect the ears from noise whenever possible. Ironically, though, when an individual begins to experience a bit of hearing loss, the typical response is to make things louder, creating a vicious cycle of ongoing damage to the hearing system. Later, we will see how the various elements of the Save Your Hearing Now Program protect the ears from noise-related damage, and very likely slow damage caused by the aging process as well.

Drugs That Harm Our Hearing

Minimizing the noise levels in daily life is one way to protect hearing. As I mention in Chapter Three, avoiding certain medications is another important factor. Recent headlines have underscored the potentially serious health risks linked to a number of prescription medications, including tremendously popular pain relievers like Crestor, Celebrex, Vioxx, Bextra, and Vicodin. In fact, adverse drug reactions cause about 100,000 deaths in this country each year, while drug recalls and revised, stricter warnings on pharmaceuticals have become regular events.

Certainly, dangerous side effects and drug reactions are important news. But where are the headlines about drug-related hearing loss? The truth is that few physicians warn patients that the medication they are being given could affect hearing. And as we saw in Jackie's example, even common, over-the-counter drugs, like aspirin and other NSAIDs, may take a toll.

Are doctors being irresponsible? Not really. Drugs can affect people differently, so there's no way for a physician to know that one patient will be fine while another may experience hearing loss. Another difficulty here is that side effects from many drugs don't occur instantly. As the drug accumulates in the body, a process that can take weeks or months, an individual may start to experience side effects, but not connect them with the drug she or he has been taking.

Ototoxic drugs may cause hearing loss in an individual with normal hearing, or worsen existing hearing loss. Hundreds of drugs fall into the ototoxic category (for a list see page 44). Reactions involving these drugs can be temporary, in which case hearing returns to normal sometime after the drug is stopped, but drugs may cause permanent hearing damage.

Clearly, the link between drugs and hearing loss poses a tremendous problem for many people who do not have the luxury of doing without or switching to a less harmful remedy. And no one should ever—I repeat, *ever*—stop taking medication abruptly because of hearing loss concerns. If you suspect your hearing is being affected by medication, discuss the situation with your physician. In many cases, there are alternatives available.

When options don't exist, the Save Your Hearing Now Program can support hearing and provide protection against the erosion caused by some drugs. The supplement recommendations in this book should be discussed with your physician or a health care provider who is knowledgeable about drug-supplement interactions. In the case of chemotherapeutic agents, for example, certain antioxidants may not be compatible and should not be taken concurrently, but could be used once the chemotherapy ends.

Another way to approach the drug dilemma is to ask your doctor before starting a new prescription whether the drug is likely to affect hearing and if there are less ototoxic alternatives. If your doctor doesn't know, don't be surprised. Ask him to do a little detective work, or check with your pharmacist. If the options are limited, don't despair. Since the same drug can affect two people very differently, hearing damage is not necessarily a given.

If hearing loss is a possible side effect of the medication your physician is prescribing, it makes sense to monitor that drug's specific impact on hearing. Ideally, an audiologist should conduct tests before beginning medication to obtain a baseline. Those tests should be repeated several times during the course of treatment. Normally, an audiologist checks hearing in the 250 to 8,000 Hz range, but to monitor drug-related hearing loss, it is best to examine the high-frequency range (between 9,000 and 20,000 Hz), where damage is likely to occur first. If hearing is being affected, the prescribing physician may be able to recommend a safer alternative before your usable hearing is wiped out.

Other Causes of Hearing Loss

There are literally dozens of types of hearing loss. As we have seen, it may be temporary or occur gradually. Hearing loss can affect one or both ears. In addition, it can be permanent, sudden, or temporary. Most often, the cause of the problem is obvious, but there are instances when hearing loss cannot be explained.

One of the most common sources of hearing problems is accumulated earwax. This is easily remedied by a physician, although some people prefer the do-it-yourself method. In this case, it's best to follow your doctor's instructions (or see page 13 for my advice on how to remove earwax). Under no circumstances should you insert cotton swabs, cotton balls, or other foreign objects into the ear to remove earwax. Swabs, sticks, and the like can rupture the eardrum, an event that demands immediate medical attention.

Here are some other types of hearing loss:

A benign tumor that develops on the auditory nerve, *acoustic neuroma* (or *vestibular schwannoma*), may affect hearing, as well as sense of balance. Most commonly, acoustic neuromas are found in adults and are the most common benign growth in the internal auditory canal inside the brain. The most common symptoms are ringing in one ear, and there may also be hearing loss in that ear. Anyone who experiences one-sided ringing/buzzing with or without hearing loss should schedule an appointment with an otolaryngologist/head and neck surgeon or ENT.

A bacterial infection of the middle ear, *otitis media*, may affect hearing by allowing fluids to gather. Infection can also damage the eardrum or, in severe cases erode a portion of the inner ear bones. Antibiotics used to be the first line of treatment for ear infections, but there are new ways of dealing with this all-too-common problem, which we look at in Chapter Twelve.

Subjecting the ears to intense broadband noise (i.e., not an isolated frequency, but a range of frequencies, such as from 1 to 4 kHz) can create a condition known as *boilermaker's ear.* A loud assembly line is a good example of broadband noise.

Although it is not technically a loss of hearing ability, *hyperacusis* is an often devastating disorder that begins with a damaged cochlea. The end result is a perceived amplification of sounds to intolerable levels, so that ordinary sounds become painful. Often, tinnitus, a condition that involves ringing, buzzing, or hissing sounds (see below), also occurs with hyperacusis.

Somewhere between 3 and 5 million people suffer from the disorienting condition known as *Ménière's disease.* Dizziness, difficulty hearing, tinnitus, and ear pressure (or fullness) are common symptoms. The cause, however, remains elusive, as does a remedy. (You can read more about Ménière's disease in Chapter Thirteen.)

Otosclerosis occurs when the stirrup or stapes bone (the

smallest bone in the body) develops a bony overgrowth and prevents the movement necessary to relay vibrations to the brain. This is often a hereditary condition, and for reasons that are not known, it tends to occur most frequently in older women of Caucasian descent. Technically, it is a type of conductive hearing loss and is treated with surgery, which is often quite successful at returning hearing to normal levels.

Sudden sensorineural hearing loss is a real medical mystery. Although it is thought to be related to a virus or a vascular problem, this rare condition—which affects roughly four thousand Americans annually—generally appears in only one ear. Some literature suggests a 50 to 60 percent chance of spontaneous recovery, but in my own experience, the figure is lower. If treated rapidly with steroids, antivirals, and/or medications to enhance blood flow, a certain amount of hearing can sometimes be recovered.

Tinnitus is a widespread disorder, characterized by sometimes maddening levels of buzzing, hissing, or ringing sounds. Reported by more than 80 percent of all individuals with hearing loss, tinnitus may be a constant or intermittent experience. Not long ago, tinnitus was attributed to damage within the ear, but now it is believed to begin in the brain, often in response to ototoxic medications or exposure to loud sounds. Tinnitus is still a bit of a mystery, but current thinking is that the brain is trying to overcome damage to the ears' sensory cells by creating its own electrical signals, which cause noise. (See Chapter Twelve for a more detailed look at tinnitus and how to treat it.)

Traumas, such as athletic or automobile accidents, explosions, shootings, or similar events, can cause tremendous damage to the ears. Ironically, air bags, which are widely considered to be lifesaving in the event of car accidents, can generate an earsplitting 170 dB or more on deployment. Drive carefully!

• • •

As you can see, the delicate workings of the auditory system are vulnerable to a wide range of factors that can diminish the ability to hear. In a sense, our ears are much like a piece of supersensitive equipment that was designed for a far quieter environment than the one we live in today. The Save Your Hearing Now Program can help reduce the amount of damage done by noise, but it is still advisable to eliminate needless, noisy activities from your life whenever possible.

((5))

FOUR STEPS TO SAVE YOUR HEARING NOW

You have seen how hearing works and understand the various factors that can cause hearing loss, as well as some ways of protecting your ears. Now let's take a look at the basics of the Save Your Hearing Now Program. There are essentially four steps involved:

1. NUTRIENTS: Take the antioxidant supplements and other nutrients that have been proven to protect against free-radical damage and enhance mitochondrial function, as well as preserve and restore hearing and enhance overall health.
2. DIET: Design meals around healthful foods that support those supplements.
3. EXERCISE: Take part in physical activity, moderately but frequently.
4. EAR PROTECTION: Avoid noise pollution whenever possible and use earplugs or other hearing protection when you are exposed to loud noise to protect the hearing abilities you have.

Step One: Nutrients

In the pages that follow, I will introduce the Save Your Hearing Now Top Ten, an all-star team of nutrients that have been scientifically proven to play vitally important roles in hearing and in slowing the aging process. In each case, there is an in-depth look at the relevant research, dosage details, and food sources of the nutrient. Typically, it is difficult—if not impossible—to obtain therapeutic amounts of these nutrients from food alone. But it is helpful to know which foods are high in key substances. In addition, many people find it helpful to see that foods they are *not* eating could be linked to hearing loss, which can be easily corrected with a dietary change or supplements. For example, vegetarians can be deficient in vitamin B_{12}, since its primary food source is meat, and vitamin B_{12} is essential for good hearing.

The effectiveness of the Save Your Hearing Now Top Ten can be enhanced with the addition of other nutrients. Most of these supporting players are not directly associated with hearing, but their importance to overall good health is well established, and in many instances, they are necessary for the proper performance of the Top Ten. You will discover why supplements are vitally important to the success of the Save Your Hearing Now Program, even for people who make an effort to eat well. Furthermore, we will explain how and when to take supplements to maximize their effectiveness.

Step Two: Diet

If the words "healthful diet" make you flinch, I'm not surprised. There is a high "yuck" factor associated with those words in our culture, because they are synonymous with deprivation. Who wants to settle down to watch the big game with a bowl of broccoli, cabbage, and carrots when a pizza or burger and fries are so quick and easy, not to mention tasty? However, poor eating habits make it difficult to get adequate nutrition, especially for older individuals. Studies have shown, for example, that a significant number of older adults fail to get amounts and types of food to meet essential energy and nutrient needs. And other research has determined that one-third of all older adults (those above the age of sixty-five) live with vitamin and mineral deficiencies.

The fact is a diet that fosters good hearing is nothing more than simple moderation and the incorporation of some key nutritional staples. And I think you will find that my recommendations are simple, doable, and proven to supply the body—and the auditory system in particular—with vital nutrients to fight hearing loss and many of the processes that occur with aging.

As with supplement suggestions, the dietary recommendations are based on carefully conducted nutritional studies published in professional journals. Instead of a fad diet or complicated eating plan, I am simply suggesting changes based on sound scientific evidence. There is a wide range of foods to choose from. Many are recommended because they are excellent sources of free-radical-fighting antioxidants, while others support the work of the supplements or provide additional benefits related to hearing.

Step Three: Exercise

A sedentary lifestyle is on the verge of eclipsing smoking in terms of the number of deaths it causes. If that's not enough to get you off the couch, there are three reasons why your hearing will benefit from moderate workouts. One, exercise stimulates circulation throughout the body, which is very important for a healthy auditory system, as well as for cardiovascular health.

In fact, just about everything that keeps the heart healthy also helps hearing, because both systems thrive with the elements in the Save Your Hearing Now Program. Two, exercise helps with weight management, and, as we will see shortly, excess weight is linked to accelerated aging, along with a host of other health problems, most of which harm hearing. Three, people who are having problems hearing are often suffering from depression or stress. Exercise is a proven method of combating both stress and depression without causing the unwanted and potentially dangerous side effects linked to pharmaceutical remedies. If you start getting regular moderate exercise, you will very likely find that you have more energy, sleep better, and have an overall improvement in mood. You will also be supporting the work of the antioxidants that protect hearing.

Trust me, exercise does not have to be a chore, and sore muscles are not inevitable. There are many ways to make exercise enjoyable and effective.

Step Four: Ear Protection

Our noisy world makes ear protection an essential part of the Save Your Hearing Now Program. Of course, factors like lifestyle, occupation, age, hobbies, and the present condition of your hearing have to be considered, too. But seldom do I see a patient who couldn't benefit from some type of ear protection.

Fortunately, the technology involved in ear protection has improved greatly, so there are a number of new choices available in earplugs and earmuffs that are far superior to earlier models. It is now possible, for example, to wear ear protection and still have a fairly normal conversation in a noisy environment. And we will also look at various ways to give the ears "quiet time," an important element that allows the hair cells to relax and heal.

Before You Start

Before beginning the program, it is essential to recognize that the information in this book is not meant to substitute for a medical evaluation by a trained professional. Only an experienced physician familiar with your individual situation can decide what measures are right for you. If you have been sedentary or are being treated for any health condition, discuss this program with your physician beforehand and obtain his or her approval. In addition, if you are experiencing hearing loss, it would be wise to have your hearing tested by a reputable, independent audiologist or at your ENT/surgeon's office to get a baseline reading. Some individuals notice that hearing loss stabilizes fairly quickly; others find that certain types of sounds, such as conversations or television programs, are clearer or easier to hear.

As you become familiar with the program in the following pages, remember that no two people are alike; we all process supplements and food differently, and our bodies don't respond to exercise in the same way. It is important to maintain reasonable expectations and allow your auditory system sufficient time to heal. Understand that a nutrient-based program does not work overnight. Many people, accustomed to taking an aspirin and experiencing pain relief, are disappointed with anything that doesn't provide instant results. Keep in mind, though, that the aspirin is simply masking the symptoms of the headache, not correcting the cause. The Save Your Hearing Now Program works by rebuilding and defending cells throughout the body, particularly in the auditory system. The damage didn't happen overnight, and the repair work takes time, too.

Finally, please don't stress out over the inevitable slips— the occasional not-so-healthful meal, or the weekend away when you forgot the supplements. The Save Your Hearing Now Program isn't about being perfect or setting impossibly high standards. It's designed to improve your hearing and health simultaneously. So let's get started!

(((6)))

STEP ONE: THE NUTRIENTS YOU NEED

Whenever the subject of vitamins and other nutritional supplements comes up, someone invariably asks, "If I eat well, why do I need to take vitamins?"

There is plenty of proof that vitamins play a valuable role in good health. Not long ago, a survey conducted by the Lewin Group found that if all adults simply took a daily multivitamin, Americans could save $1.6 billion in health care costs by reducing the risk of coronary artery disease and improving immune system functions. In spite of that, supplements remain a controversial subject, even in the medical profession. But here is my take on the issue: Very few of us, myself included, "eat well" all the time. Furthermore, even when we do eat well, it's impossible to be certain how much, if any, nutrition is in the food we are eating.

Consider the mineral magnesium, for example. Among other things, magnesium is essential for a healthy cardiovascular system and strong bones. It also activates enzymes throughout the body, oversees metabolism, promotes proper nerve functions and muscle contractions, and is involved in insulin production as well as aiding blood sugar management in people with diabetes. Magnesium also has a little-known but strong link to good hearing.

We don't need a great deal of magnesium; the recommended daily allowance (RDA) for adults is only 400 milligrams (mg). In spite of that, a study conducted by the U.S. Department of Agriculture (USDA) determined that a whopping 75 percent of Americans are getting insufficient amounts of magnesium from the food they eat. Not surprisingly, processed foods, which are typically low in the mineral, are partly to blame. But farmland in this country has largely been drained of magnesium, too, so even a diet that includes magnesium-rich foods (nuts, legumes, potatoes, green leafy vegetables) may not be enough to maintain adequate levels of the nutrient.

Still not convinced? For the sake of argument, let's say you do eat well and your food is grown in high-quality soil, so it's loaded with nutrients. Do you avoid all over-the-counter and prescription medications, including antibiotics? Do you live in an area that is not polluted by noise or toxic substances? (Probably not, since noise is widespread and toxins have even been found within the Arctic Circle.) Is your life free of stress? Do you engage in moderate physical activity for at least thirty minutes on most days of the week? Do you eat primarily lightly cooked, whole, organic food? If your answer to even one of these questions is no, then you probably need more nutrition than you're getting from food.

To me, the real issue isn't whether or not you should take supplements, but *which* supplements you should take and in what doses. Here's why: Combating free-radical damage requires more of certain substances, especially antioxidants and the nutrients that support them. A multivitamin is better than nothing, but building on that foundation with other compounds that have been proven effective is an even better way to go.

One more thing: Many people complain about the high cost of vitamins. Let's put this in perspective. Health care costs in this country are rising at a far higher pace than incomes. In fact, a survey by the Center for Studying Health System Change found an 8.2 percent increase in consumer spending on physician services, hospital care, and pharmaceuticals in 2004. The year before, the rise was 8.4 percent. To make matters worse, employers are increasingly cutting back on health care benefits, leaving employees to shoulder more of the expense.[1] So while it may seem that cutting-edge vitamins are a somewhat costly luxury, they are barely a blip on a budget compared to the expense of a hospital visit. All-natural, bioavailable supplements in a patented formula do cost more than run-of-the-mill versions. But generally, the bargain-priced products are poorly absorbed and tend to provide dosages that are either too low to have health benefits or in a synthetic form that the body does not recognize.

Finally, studies have repeatedly shown the extensive health benefits that can be obtained from supplements. For example, researchers at Johns Hopkins University found a reduced risk of Alzheimer's disease in elderly individuals who took a combination of vitamins C and E or a multivitamin containing vitamin C.[2] Meanwhile, a study from Dallas's Cooper Institute found lower levels of C-reactive protein, a substance associated with an increased risk of both heart disease and diabetes, in individuals who took multivitamins.[3] And multivitamins have been shown to enhance immunity, making the body better able to withstand assaults by bacteria and virus.[4]

ARE MEDICATIONS ROBBING YOUR BODY'S NUTRIENTS?

One of the less advertised side effects of prescription medicines is that they frequently rob the body of nutrients, including many vitamins, minerals, and related compounds. Take aspirin, for example. Popping a couple of aspirin on a regular basis can lead to hearing loss. But that's not all. Aspirin also reduces levels of vitamin C, calcium, folic acid, iron, potassium, sodium, and vitamin B_5.

Here's another example. Oral contraceptives, the birth control pills regularly taken by millions of women, lower supplies of folic acid, vitamins B_1, B_2, B_3, B_6, B_{12}, and C, as well as magnesium, selenium, and zinc. And cholesterol-lowering statins rob the body of CoQ10, a nutrient now considered essential for heart health! Naturally, with decreased stores of hearing-supportive nutrients, antioxidants, and minerals, hearing could very well be affected.

Don't panic, though, because this does not mean you have to give up the medication. (And *never* abruptly stop taking medication without first consulting your physician, even if you think your hearing is being affected.) If you know what nutrients you're likely to be lacking, simply take supplements and eat more foods with those substances to make up for the loss. Your physician may be able to advise you, and here are a couple of books that can help: *Drug-Induced Nutrient Depletion Handbook,* from Lexi-Comp's Clinical Reference Library is written by a panel of pharmacists and updated annually. *The Nutritional Cost of Prescription Drugs: How to Maintain Good Nutrition While Using Prescription Drugs,* by Ross Pelton, R.Ph., and James B. LaValle, R.Ph. (Morton Publishing, 2000), covers much of the same ground as the first book, but in a more consumer-friendly fashion.

Some physicians still insist that people with low stress levels who consume a healthful diet, including five to ten helpings of fruits and vegetables a day, do not need nutritional supplements. It is clear, however, that most of the American population—most of the world population, for that matter—does not adhere to that regimen.

As I noted earlier, there is a considerable body of evidence demonstrating that the average person can benefit significantly from nutritional supplements. For individuals with hearing loss, it appears that supplements are even more essential. As we have seen, the most common types of hearing loss are signs of free-radical damage. Certainly, the free-radicals are not just attacking the ears; the same injuries are occurring in cells throughout the body. Supplements are a simple, effective way of giving the body the tools it needs to protect itself.

HOW VITAMINS CAN HELP HEARING

When it came to vitamins, Frances was not interested. She felt fine, ate a well-balanced diet, and simply didn't see why she should spend good money on something that she felt had no benefits.

Then her daughter, Marcia, became engaged. As the wedding planning intensified, Frances found herself growing so anxious that she had trouble eating, sleeping, and concentrating. On top of it all, it was difficult for her to hear conversations, so she had to ask people to repeat everything. "It was, according to my husband, like watching a train wreck in slow motion. Trying to help Marcia plan the event, choose a gown, arrange the reception, and manage all those details was completely unnerving. Not being able to hear properly wasn't helping, either."

Finally, a friend became concerned. She suggested Frances ask her doctor for a shot of vitamin B_{12}, which, the friend explained, had gotten her through an emotionally difficult time. After considerable urging by her family, Frances agreed. That shot, she now says, changed her attitude toward vitamins completely.

"I could not believe what a difference it made," she recalls. "Night and day. I went into the doctor's office feeling like I was going to either burst into tears at any second or bite someone's head off. Then, seemingly just seconds after he gave me the shot, I felt like a normal human being again. All that tension and anxiety just went away."

When Frances remarked on how different she felt, the doctor explained that vitamin B_{12} deficiencies are not uncommon among older people, because the nutrient can be difficult to absorb in later years, and the average diet typically does not provide enough of many of the nutrients we need. Since many of the symptoms of a B_{12} deficiency are similar to those seen in dementia patients, they can be misread as signs of aging.

The next week, Frances returned to the doctor with Marcia in tow, and during the following months, they rarely missed their B_{12} injections. The wedding was a huge success, but Frances is the first to admit that she and her daughter would never have made it through the event without the B_{12} shots. Now that her life and her hearing have returned to normal, Frances is exploring nutrients that go beyond a simple multivitamin/mineral supplement, "just to be on the safe side," she explains. "There's a grandchild on the way, and I'm planning on being able to hear his first words."

Vitamins 101

Vitamins are substances that are essential to proper functioning of the human body. In fact, a substance is considered a vitamin if we develop a disease without it. Scurvy, for example, is caused by a lack of vitamin C, which the human body cannot manufacture.

Vitamins are classified as either water-soluble or fat-soluble. All members of the vitamin B family are water-soluble, as is vitamin C. The others—vitamin A, D, and E—are fat-soluble. The kidneys filter and process water-soluble vitamins, and they are then excreted from the body in the urine. Because they are not stored in the body, we need to replenish stores of water-soluble vitamins. On the other hand, fat-soluble vitamins can be stored in body fat and accessed as necessary. This is a bit of a double-edged sword, though, because high doses of fat-soluble vitamins can accumulate and reach toxic levels with prolonged intake, something that does not happen with water-soluble vitamins.

Standard multivitamins provide both water- and fat-soluble nutrients, including well-known antioxidants, like vitamins C and E. In addition to vitamins, the body also needs minerals to perform properly. The best known of these is probably calcium, which has received a great deal of attention because of its connection to strong bones. But lesser-known minerals, like boron, magnesium, manganese, copper, molybdenum, selenium, and zinc, for example, support the work of various vitamins and perform other critical functions, some of which are involved in hearing, cardiovascular health, circulation, and aging. Frequently, these nutrients are primarily found in foods that few people eat, so clearly, the best way to obtain them is with a mineral supplement.

If you're taking a multivitamin-mineral supplement, you're creating the foundation for better hearing. But there's so much more that can be done. The Save Your Hearing Now Program's Top Ten nutrient list is the best place to begin. The foundation rests on four substances, ALA (alpha-lipoic acid) and acetyl-L-carnitine (ALC), the two compounds that were the focus of my earliest research on hearing loss prevention and nutrients—and two other potent antioxidants, coenzyme Q10 and glutathione. In combination, these four compounds deliver state-of-the-art protection for the auditory system. An additional six other nutrients round out the program.

The complete Save Your Hearing Now Top Ten list:

1. **ALA:** A powerful and versatile antioxidant, ALA is capable of counteracting the type of free-radical damage that harms the auditory system.

   Recommended dosage: 100 to 750 mg per day

2. **ALC:** This compound is important for the proper functioning of the mitochondria, as well as supporting a healthy nervous system and brain, where much of the auditory system is located.

   Recommended dosage: 500 to 3,000 mg per day

3. **Glutathione:** A key element in preventing free-radical damage that can harm hearing, glutathione also minimizes the effects of various pollutants.

   Recommended dosage: 30 to 300 mg per day

4. **Coenzyme Q10 (CoQ10):** This vitally important antioxidant protects the mitochondria—and therefore hearing—and also plays a role in the production of cellular energy.

   Recommended dosage: 60 to 320 mg per day

5. **Vitamin B complex:** A family of nutrients that perform literally hundreds of tasks in the body, vitamin B has a special affinity for the nervous system and hearing.

   Recommended dosage: a balanced formula containing the entire family in appropriate amounts

6. **Lecithin:** This substance is essential for healthy cell membranes, and my own research has shown that it protects against hearing loss.

   Recommended dosage: 200 to 1,500 mg per day

7. **N-acetylcysteine (NAC):** An amino acid known best for its ability to detoxify, NAC has also been shown to repair damaged hair cells of the inner ear.

   Recommended dosage: 100 to 2,500 mg per day

8. **Quercetin:** A bioflavonoid found in fruits and vegetables, quercetin has antioxidant properties that make it a powerful antidote to free-radical damage that can destroy hearing.

   Recommended dosage: 30 to 500 mg per day

9. **Resveratrol:** This compound, found in red wine, grape juice, and grapes, is considered a potent antiaging weapon.

   Recommended dosage: 40 to 1,000 mg per day

10. **Zinc:** The mineral zinc is an important antioxidant involved in hundreds of processes throughout the body, including support of the immune system. The highest concentrations of zinc are found in the inner ear and in the eye, and it is involved in hearing.

    Recommended dosage: 15 to 75 mg per day

For best absorption, these supplements should be taken with food and at least eight ounces of water. I recommend separating the daily dose you choose into two or three portions—whatever works best for you—so that your cells are nourished throughout the day.

Because these elements are widely recognized as powerful substances that affect various aspects of health, they are at the center of the Save Your Hearing Now Program. Yes, it is revolutionary to use a nutrient-based approach to protecting the auditory system. But scientists are increasingly discovering that vitamins, minerals, and related compounds have significant healing properties throughout the body. The Save Your Hearing Now Program combines nutrients known to support healthy hearing into a safe, effective regimen. When used in conjunction with the program's three other aspects— healthful diet, physical activity, and hearing protection—the results can be dramatic.

As you can see, most of these substances are not typically included in a multivitamin/mineral formula, and others, such as NAC, are not found in food. Still, there is a considerable body of research showing that these compounds are vitally important to protecting various aspects of the auditory system. Let's look at each one of these nutrients in depth, to see why and how they are important to the Save Your Hearing Now Program.

Putting the Power of ALA and ALC to Work

In Chapter Three, we looked at the link between the common aging deletion, which damages the mitochondria, the tiny energy factories within each cell, and mitochondrial damage. The common aging deletion is thought to be responsible for hearing loss, the aging process, and a long list of other disorders. Studies have shown that when the mitochondria are damaged, energy production in cells slows down and the cells may even die. As mitochondrial damage accumulates over the years, the body begins to show signs of aging. Hearing loss is one of those signs. As you may recall, in my research with antioxidants, I was able to show that both ALA (alpha-lipoic acid) and ALC (acetyl-L-carnitine), as well as several other substances, can slow, stop, and even reverse the damage that results during aging and hearing loss.

Individually, ALA and ALC do an outstanding job of fighting free radicals, but when they are combined, the synergy that results puts them in a league of their own. Adding

CoQ10 and glutathione to the mix boosts their effectiveness even more. Hundreds of studies show why these four substances are the foundation of the Save Your Hearing Now Program's supplement recommendations. But ALA, ALC, CoQ10, and glutathione can do far more than protect hearing.

ALA

Alpha-lipoic acid (ALA) is a vitamin-like substance that is essential for proper energy production in our cells, among other important things. You can get small amounts of ALA from organ meats and green leafy vegetables, but not enough to do much good.

ALA hasn't received as much publicity as some nutrients, like vitamins C and E. But scientists consider it a very powerful antioxidant. Not long ago, University of California, Berkeley, researcher Lester Packer, Ph.D., an internationally recognized expert on ALA (he's published sixty-some papers on the substance), was interviewed on *World News Tonight with Peter Jennings*. Dr. Packer described ALA as quite possibly the most effective naturally occurring antioxidant that's been discovered thus far.[5]

A truly versatile substance, ALA can be used to:

- Decrease damage to the heart caused by heart attacks[6]
- Treat diabetic-induced nerve dysfunction (neuropathy)[7]
- Regulate glucose metabolism and insulin function in diabetics[8]
- Treat various types of liver damage, including that caused by cirrhosis, hepatitis C, and poison mushrooms[9]
- Interrupt viral activation and cell death that occurs in HIV patients[10]
- "Recycle" vitamins C and E, so that they remain in the body longer[11]

ALC

Like ALA, ALC (also known as ALCAR), a derivative of the amino acid L-carnitine, is produced in the body. As with other nutrients, production slows as we age. And since meat and animal products are the best food sources of the nutrient, vegetarians and vegans may have a difficult time getting enough ALC at any age.

Before going on, let's clarify one important point. It is important not to confuse acetyl-L-carnitine with L-carnitine, even though they are closely related. L-carnitine can be utilized by the muscles, but it doesn't cross the blood-brain barrier very well, and so is not likely to reach the ear. But acetyl-L-carnitine, or ALC, is a different story. It is much more "bioavailable," which is simply the scientific term for substances that have no trouble reaching cells within the brain and ears.

Part of ALC's "day job" is to relay valuable fatty acids from cells to the mitochondria for energy production. There have been literally dozens of studies with ALC; by and large, these show that the substance increases longevity, enhances cardiac performance and learning abilities, and improves depression and Alzheimer's symptoms in the elderly. It has also shown promise in treating diabetic neuropathy and HIV.[12]

In addition, my earlier research with ALC has new support from a study at the Hough Ear Institute in Oklahoma City. Both ALC and N-acetylcysteine (NAC), a compound that we look at in more detail later in this chapter, were shown to significantly reduce noise-related damage to the cochlea's hair cells, and thereby protect hearing.[13]

ALA and ALC: Synergy Happens

All in all, these two supplements are impressive performers, especially when it comes to improving hearing and slowing the aging process. But there's something else that sets ALA and ALC apart. We hear a great deal these days about "synergy," the enhanced results that occur when we put one and one together and end up with three (or sometimes even four or five). In recent years, a number of antiaging studies have looked at the benefits of ALA and ALC individually and combined. In most cases, the combination is synergistic. In other words, more benefits are generated by using both supplements at the same time than by using one or the other alone.

This dynamic duo was prominently featured in the media recently, when researchers used a combination of ALA and ALC to create a veritable "fountain of youth." In laboratories at the University of California, Berkeley, and the Linus Pauling Institute at Oregon State University, elderly rats were divided into two groups. One segment was given a combination of ALA and ALC, while the other group (used as a control) received no supplements.

After only one month, the supplemented rats were twice as active as those in the control group. In fact, in terms of activity level, these rats could pass for middle-aged animals. In addition to increased metabolism, the treated rats had other advantages: Their memory and thinking abilities were much better than the control group's, they had less free-radical damage at the cellular level, and the supplements even protected their hearts from the aging process. In other words, the combined benefits of ALA and ALC were substantially greater than the individual abilities they had demonstrated in earlier research.[14] As you may recall, we had similar results in our research with rats and hearing loss.

The results of this study, funded by the National Institutes of Aging (NIA) and reported in the *Proceedings of the National Academy of Sciences* journal and *Annals of the New York Academy of Science*, were deemed so exciting that human clinical trials began almost immediately.

Because of the growing body of scientific research supporting the benefits of these two substances, ALA and ALC are now widely available in supplement form. They can be found individually and combined from various manufacturers. (See page 236 in Resources.)

THE OTHER HALF OF THE FANTASTIC FOUR

While ALA and ALC are undoubtedly important, I believe their function is further strengthened by combining them with CoQ10 and glutathione. Let me explain how these two substances protect and preserve hearing, too.

Although it is not technically a vitamin, CoQ10 is considered a potent, fat-soluble antioxidant with a special ability to protect the mitochondria, which makes it vitally important to good hearing. It has also been shown to preserve hearing in individuals who were experiencing hearing loss due to mutations of the mitochondria.[15]

Found in cells throughout the body, CoQ10 plays a significant role in heart health and immunity. In fact, research with both animals and humans has demonstrated CoQ10's ability to strengthen the heart, reduce the formation of LDL ("bad") cholesterol, enhance circulation, fight aging, and help reduce high blood pressure. A number of studies have shown that it is highly effective at combating free radicals, and it also has the ability to "recycle" vitamins C and E after these antioxidants have been damaged by encounters with free radicals.

Although our bodies produce CoQ10, production slows considerably as we age. As far as food sources, CoQ10 is found in beef, fatty types of seafood (salmon and sardines), peanuts, wheat germ, rice bran, soy oil, and organ meats. Levels of CoQ10 in food are low, however, and cooking destroys most of this vital substance.

Signs of insufficient CoQ10 levels include fatigue, diabetes, and gum disease. It's also important to note that cholesterol-lowering statins deplete the body's CoQ10 stores, as do tricyclic antidepressants, anticoagulants, and the blood pressure medication known as beta-blockers.

As for glutathione, this versatile antioxidant shields cells from free radicals and works in conjunction with other antioxidants to protect the liver, the cardiovascular and immune systems, brain, and skin from damage by these rogue molecules, making it a useful age-fighter. It also helps eliminate environmental toxins from the body.

Research has shown that glutathione can protect against both noise-induced hearing loss and the damage caused to hearing by a common chemotherapy drug.[16]

There is some question as to how well the body absorbs glutathione supplements, which is why I recommend the more absorbable form, known as glutathione ethyl ester. Furthermore, a related compound, NAC (see below), also enhances glutathione's bioavailability.

Glutathione is found in some foods, including avocado, grapefruit, watermelon, potatoes, asparagus, strawberries, oranges, tomatoes, broccoli, and zucchini. Supplements, however, are the most consistent method for providing your body with a regular supply of this important nutrient.

For adequate hearing benefits, I suggest aiming for a dosage of 100 to 750 mg per day of ALA, and 500 to 3,000 mg of ALC, 60 to 320 mg of CoQ10, and 30 to 300 mg of glutathione. ALA and ALC can be very energizing, as a number of patients have reported. For that reason, some people prefer to take them in the morning and at midday, while others take them in the morning and evening. You may want to experiment to see how taking them at different times of day affects you.

The proof that ALA, ALC, CoQ10, and glutathione can

protect hearing in humans has been amply demonstrated by any number of glowing reports from patients. Ivan's story is a good example. After years of working as a baggage handler at a major airport, Ivan's hearing was deteriorating quickly, even though he always wore sufficient ear protection on the job. His family life was suffering because of the hearing loss. Frustrated by his inability to hear well, Ivan's wife and children were threatening to stop speaking to him if he didn't get a hearing aid. But the price of a good hearing aid was an obstacle at the moment, so Ivan came to see me, wondering if there was something else he could do.

I recommended Ivan start taking ALA, ALC, CoQ10, and glutathione along with the other nutrients on the program. At first, he was reluctant. "I already take vitamins," he said, "and they aren't helping." I explained how these four ingredients are different and how my own research had proven that they could protect the ears. Then, as we continued the examination, I discovered that Ivan's father and several uncles had all suffered from hearing loss, which indicated that genetics probably played a role.

"Do any of your children have hearing problems?" I asked.

"Well, my son, Daniel, is not doing very well at school, and the teacher says it's because he doesn't listen."

I strongly recommended that Daniel have his hearing tested, which was done the following week. Not surprisingly, the eleven-year-old was also experiencing hearing loss. He, too, began taking a supplement that included the four recommended substances. In addition, I suggested that his teacher be advised of his condition, so that changes could be made in the classroom for him. We also discussed various methods of protecting the ears from noise.

Not long afterward, I heard from both Ivan and Daniel. The boy was doing much better at school and felt that his hearing was actually improving. Ivan, however, wasn't sure that anything had changed. He was still having a hard time at home and was ready to throw in the towel. As we continued to talk, though, I discovered that Ivan was taking the same amount of ALA, ALC, CoQ10, and glutathione as Daniel, even though he was easily twice the boy's size. "Why don't you increase your supplement dosage somewhat," I suggested, "and see if that makes a difference?"

In spite of his doubts, Ivan did so, and the next time I heard from him, things had improved considerably. He felt that his hearing was no longer getting steadily worse. Ivan also found that conversations at home were improving. "As long as the television isn't on, my family doesn't have to shout at me, so we turn it off at dinnertime and when we want to talk," he explained.

Meanwhile, Daniel was becoming a star pupil. "All this time, they thought he had a learning disability, but he was just having problems hearing," Ivan reported. "Now he's doing great."

Ivan and Daniel aren't the only people who have had successful experiences with ALA, ALC, CoQ10, and glutathione. When it comes to protecting hearing, however, these four substances are part of the story. There are many other nutrients that support their activity and have benefits that extend beyond improved hearing. Let's look at the six additional nutrients that make up the Save Your Hearing Now Top Ten.

DECIPHERING THE RECOMMENDED DAILY ALLOWANCE (RDA)

The typical multivitamin usually includes vitamins A, B complex, C, D, and E, but the quantities of these nutrients in the formula may be lower than the recommended daily (or Dietary) allowance (RDA). The product label provides details on what percentage of RDA the product contains, so you can see how much of each nutrient each pill provides.

The RDAs were first established by the Food and Nutrition Board in 1941, and they are updated from time to time. They are considered the best scientific advice on nutritional needs and are designed to be appropriate for nearly all healthy people.

While the RDAs are widely believed to be safe levels, keep in mind that they are neither minimal requirements nor optimal levels. Many nutrition experts believe that our current vitamin and mineral guidelines are inadequate for promoting good health.

Adequate intake (AI) is another term sometimes used in dosage recommendations. This means that more studies need to be conducted to determine the nutrient's RDA, but in the meantime the suggested dosage is based on our current scientific knowledge of its role in maintaining good health.

Vitamin B Complex

The incredibly versatile and essential nutrients that make up the vitamin B complex play a huge role in hearing health because they are critical for proper functioning of nerves throughout the body. Because the B vitamins need one another to function properly, they are typically taken together in a combination formula, either as a separate nutrient or as an ingredient in a multivitamin. If your multivitamin has fairly low levels of B complex, such as no more than 10 mg of the "large-dose Bs" (those in which dosage recommendations are listed in milligrams, or mg, such as B_1, B_2, B_3, and so on, rather than micrograms, or mcg), it makes sense to take an additional balanced B complex supplement. These are usually identified by the number of milligrams in the large-dose Bs, so the label might read "B Complex—20," "B Complex—50," or "B Complex—100."

Not only is this family of substances widely used throughout the body for hundreds of basic functions, but specific B vitamins are also linked to hearing (B_{12}) and heart health (folate, B_6, and B_{12}), which means they are also important for good hearing.

Since they are water-soluble, the B vitamins are not stored in the body's tissues, so supplies need to be replenished on a daily basis. Unfortunately, Americans do not seem to be getting sufficient amounts of B vitamins. Vitamin B_6 deficiency, for example, is quite common in this country. In fact, a report from the U.S. Department of Agriculture (USDA) found that a stunning 80 percent of all Americans are getting less than the recommended daily allowance (RDA) of this nutrient. Part of the problem is that cooking and food processing reduce vitamin B_6 content in food. Here is a closer look at this very important group of nutrients:

B_1: Thiamine

The first B vitamin to be identified, B_1 performs a long list of tasks in the body, including maintaining a regular heartbeat, supporting metabolism of amino acids and carbohydrates, and keeping the brain functioning at optimal levels. B_1 also serves as an antioxidant and plays a role in glucose absorption. It also helps with the energy production process in the cells.

A deficiency of vitamin B_1 is responsible for beriberi, a nerve disease that is seldom seen in the civilized world these days. In addition, inadequate B_1 can result in fatigue, constipation, tingling or numbness in the extremities, and muscle problems, including soreness.

Low levels of B_1 are typically found in people who consume excessive amounts of alcohol, take antibiotics or oral contraceptives, or eat a diet of poor-quality, highly processed foods.

DOSAGE: The RDA is 1.1 mg for women and 1.2 mg for men. Doses as high as 100 mg per day are considered safe.

FOODS: Brown rice, wheat germ, whole grains, egg yolks, oysters, green peas, black beans, legumes, fish, and foods that are enriched with selected B vitamins (check the labels on cereal, pasta, and bread) are good sources.

B_2: Riboflavin

B_2, another antioxidant, is involved in a number of cellular processes and in metabolism, and also plays a role in fighting depression. B_2 helps keep the eyes, skin, hair, and fingernails strong and healthy and is essential for the production of red blood cells.

A deficiency of B_2 might manifest itself in skin problems such as dry skin, cracked lips, or cracked skin in the corners of the mouth. Other symptoms of too little B_2 include hair loss, depression, sensitivity to light, sleep problems, and digestive disorders.

Heavy drinking, birth control pills, antibiotics, some chemotherapeutic agents, and intense workouts can all rob the body of B_2.

DOSAGE: The RDA is 1.1 mg for women and 1.3 mg for men. Doses as high as 100 mg per day are considered safe.

Foods: Milk and other dairy products, meat and liver, egg yolks, whole grains, spinach, avocado, brewer's yeast, green leafy vegetables, and B-vitamin-enriched pasta, bread, and cereal are all good sources.

B₃: Niacin

Enhanced circulation and reduced cholesterol are two benefits of niacin, which is also involved in metabolism and energy production. Like all the Bs, niacin is a true multitasker, though. It is involved in blood sugar management, digestion, hormone monitoring, and easing symptoms of adult-onset (type 2) diabetes.

Using niacin to lower cholesterol levels can be a bit tricky, though. Reducing cholesterol requires doses as high as 1,000 to 2,000 mg per day. At this level, however, "niacin flush" occurs. Niacin flush creates a warm, tingling sensation throughout the body that can last for a few seconds or as long as several hours, and some people find it an uncomfortable or even frightening experience. In addition, high doses of niacin have been linked to liver failure, even in the "nonflush" version. I advise my patients to live with the niacin flush for the cholesterol benefits, but at the same time to be careful not to exceed the suggested dosage.

Individuals who are not getting enough niacin could be at risk of developing depression, memory problems, headaches, digestive disorders, fatigue, or low blood sugar levels.

Niacin levels can be reduced by heavy drinking. Since meat and animal products are good sources of the nutrient, anyone on a vegan diet, which prohibits meat and animal products, probably needs supplements.

Dosage: The RDA is 14 mg for women and 16 mg for men.

Foods: Many foods contain niacin. Some of the richest sources are brewer's yeast, meat, poultry, and fish, legumes, organ meats, such as beef liver, milk, peanuts and peanut butter, oatmeal, and dairy products. In addition, niacin-enriched bread, pasta, and cereal are available.

B_5: Pantothenic Acid

B_5 supports the adrenal glands, so it is helpful in times of stress, depression, and anxiety. It works with other B vitamins to turn the protein, fat, and carbohydrates we eat into usable energy, and it is also a key element in the production of neurotransmitters, which relay chemical messages throughout the brain and body.

Too little pantothenic acid can cause nausea, arthritis, headache, fatigue, and acne.

DOSAGE: There is no RDA for vitamin B_5, but the "adequate intake" (AI) recommendation is 5 mg per day for both women and men. Doses up to 20 mg per day are considered safe.

FOODS: Nearly all foods contain pantothenic acid, so deficiencies are rare. Some of the best sources are brewer's yeast, beef and liver, lima beans, eggs, some fish, certain vegetables (broccoli, tomatoes, and cauliflower), nuts, legumes, and eggs.

B_6: Pyridoxine

Another hardworking member of the B family, pyridoxine is involved in more than one hundred processes related to metabolizing amino acids and protein. Vitally important to heart health, B_6, along with its cousins vitamin B_{12} and folic acid, can reduce levels of homocysteine, an amino acid with strong links to cardiovascular disease. In fact, the higher the homocysteine level, the greater the risk of heart disease.

Deficiencies of vitamin B_6 have been linked to hearing difficulties. Other symptoms include nausea and vomiting, depression, poor wound healing, cracked lips, and problems with memory.

Individuals who are taking steroids, such as cortisone, or

diuretics may not be able to absorb pyridoxine efficiently. Birth control pills, antidepressants, estrogen supplements, a high-protein diet, and heavy drinking can rob the body of pyridoxine.

DOSAGE: The RDA for both women and men is 1.3 mg.

FOODS: Vitamin B_6 is found in most foods, but as we noted above, most Americans are not getting sufficient amounts because it is destroyed in cooking and food processing. Brewer's yeast, wheat germ, peanuts and other legumes, organ meats, potatoes, spinach, sunflower seeds, and bananas are all especially rich sources of the nutrient.

B_{12}: Cyanocobalamin

In addition to helping keep the heart healthy, vitamin B_{12} is involved in cell growth and helps the brain function properly, especially in older individuals. In fact, what may appear to be dementia may actually be a deficiency of B_{12}. The nutrient also plays an important role in protecting the nerves from damage, while supporting DNA replication, and is involved in the development of healthy red blood cells.

Deficiencies of B_{12} have been linked to hearing loss (see sidebar below), as well as to depression, dizziness, memory loss, hallucinations, heart palpitations, and irritability.

Anyone who does not eat meat or animal products is at risk for a B_{12} deficiency, because the nutrient is found only in animal tissue. However, absorption problems, which are common in older individuals, could lead to inadequate levels of the nutrient in those who do consume animal products. A blood test can determine deficiencies.

DOSAGE: The RDA for both women and men is 2.4 mcg. Doses as high as 100 mcg per day are considered safe.

FOODS: B_{12} is found primarily in meat, including some seafood, and animal products (dairy and cheese), so vegetarians and vegans most likely need supplements, as do the elderly, because they may have difficulty absorbing B_{12} from food.

THE B_{12} CONNECTION TO GOOD HEARING

One of the changes that occur during aging is that digestion becomes less efficient. Nutrients from food are not easily absorbed, and this fact alone can affect hearing, as a study from the University of Georgia, Athens, demonstrates.

Researchers there discovered that older women with low blood levels of vitamin B_{12} and folate were more likely to have difficulty hearing than those with higher levels of these nutrients.[17] Since this was the first study to consider the relationship of hearing loss to vitamin intake, it needs to be replicated to verify the findings. In the meantime, of course, there is certainly no harm in getting the recommended daily dosage of B complex vitamins, which includes folate and B_{12}.

As I have noted, getting ample supplies of vitamin B_{12} can be a challenge, especially for vegetarians and vegans, older individuals, and people with anemia. Up until recently, B_{12} shots were considered the best way to increase levels of this important nutrient. But according to a new study from Israel's Rabin Medical Center, I'm happy to report that there is an alternative. After giving B_{12}-deficient patients sublingual supplements (the kind that dissolve under the tongue) of 1,000 mcg, experts found that it took only a few days for blood levels of the nutrient to reach normal levels.[18] This is especially good news for elderly people who have problems getting to a doctor's office each week, as well as those who find frequent injections uncomfortable.

Biotin

Cell growth, energy production, and carbohydrate, fat, and protein metabolism all involve the B vitamin biotin. It is also a factor in keeping hair, nails, and skin healthy, as well as protecting nerve tissue, keeping cholesterol levels down, and easing muscle aches.

Too little biotin may be responsible for eczema, depression, muscle pain, nausea, hair loss, or anemia. Since biotin is found in many foods, deficiencies are fairly rare, however.

Smoking, long courses of antibiotics, and drugs that are given to control convulsions in patients with epilepsy can deplete biotin supply. In addition, those who eat very little—either because they are dieting or because of anorexia—could have low biotin levels.

DOSAGE: There is no RDA for biotin, but the AI level is 30 mcg per day for both women and men.

FOODS: Biotin is made in the body, and it is also plentiful in animal and plant foods, such as brewer's yeast, soybeans, strawberries, peanuts, saltwater fish, watermelon, and whole grains.

Choline

The B vitamin choline plays a vital role in brain functions, because it produces a neurotransmitter known as acetylcholine, designed to relay information to the brain cells. Choline is also involved in activities in the central nervous system and helps with memory. While our bodies can produce choline, the amounts are fairly low.

High blood pressure, kidney and liver disorders, and difficulty digesting fat may occur with a choline deficiency.

Very high doses of niacin can interfere with choline absorption, even though niacin is also a B vitamin. This is why it is important to take a balanced formula, rather than individual B supplements, unless otherwise recommended by your physician.

DOSAGE: There is no RDA for choline, but the AI levels are 425 mg per day for women and 550 mg for men.

FOODS: Egg yolks are a rich source of choline, as are soybeans, peanuts and other legumes, lecithin (see below), cabbage, cauliflower, lentils, and organ meats.

Folic Acid

Cell division and the creation of cellular messengers DNA and RNA depend on adequate amounts of folic acid. This nutrient also has a well-deserved reputation for preventing birth defects and may aid in reducing symptoms of depression and anxiety. It also supports a healthy immune system, enhances brain functions, and is essential for proper formation of both white and red blood cells. In addition, folic acid is important for heart health, due to its ability to reduce homocysteine levels.

Low levels of folic acid could be responsible for anemia, problems with digestion, poor memory, fatigue, and birth defects, such as spina bifida.

Aspirin, antibiotics, antacids that contain aluminum and magnesium, birth control pills, excessive alcohol consumption, and smoking are linked to low folic acid levels.

DOSAGE: The RDA for folic acid is 400 mcg for both women and men.

FOODS: To prevent birth defects, a number of popular foods are now fortified with folic acid, including pasta, bread, and cereal. Other sources include brewer's yeast, orange juice, liver, eggs, and dark leafy vegetables, such as kale, spinach, endive, and collard greens. Cooking and microwaving these vegetables eliminates the folic acid, however, so fresh is best.

Lecithin

Technically a type of fat, lecithin is a vitally important substance when it comes to protecting hearing and keeping the heart, brain, nerves, and all the cells in the body healthy. Without this nutrient, cell walls can harden, and it becomes difficult for nutrients to enter the cell or for waste matter to be eliminated. When that happens, cells age faster than they would if the cell wall were permeable and able to function properly. For all these reasons, lecithin is essential to good hearing and minimizing the effects of aging.

Lecithin offers another advantage as well: It is a natural source of the B vitamin choline, which plays a role in proper brain functions. Studies have also shown that lecithin is useful for treating neurological conditions, such as Alzheimer's disease and bipolar disorder.

Deficiencies of lecithin are rare, since it is found in many common foods.

DOSAGE: 2 grams per day for both women and men is the average, but up to 10 grams is considered safe.

FOODS: Egg yolks, soybeans and other legumes, nuts, brewer's yeast, fish, and organ meats are all high in lecithin, but since it is used as an emulsifying agent to thicken many foods, including salad dressings, baked goods, and ice cream, it is widely available.

A CLOSER LOOK AT LECITHIN

Not long ago, my colleagues and I conducted a study with lecithin to determine its effects on hearing. The results were quite impressive. Eighteen- to twenty-month-old rats were given oral supplements of either lecithin or a placebo. We followed the subjects for six months and tested various markers of good hearing, including the common aging deletion, to determine the effect of supplements. The results showed that the lecithin-treated subjects lost approximately 12 to 15 dB of hearing, while the placebo group lost substantially more of their hearing, dropping by approximately 35 to 40 dB. In other words, lecithin provided a significant amount of protection for hearing. Furthermore, we found significantly lower production of free radicals in the lecithin group as compared to the placebo group. Mitochondrial function was significantly enhanced in the lecithin group, too, which means that the cell could produce energy in a safer, more efficient manner.[19]

N-acetylcysteine (NAC)

Ignore the industrial-sounding name and make friends with the amino acid derivative N-acetylcysteine (NAC), especially if you're interested in protecting against noise-related damage to the cochlea's hair cells. A Swedish study found that NAC's antioxidant capabilities reduced hair cell loss during exposure to loud noises, and NAC provided as much protection as ALC in a similar study in the United States.[20]

The cardiovascular system can benefit from NAC, too; it has been linked to reductions in homocysteine and lipoprotein(a), two substances considered risk factors for heart disease. Furthermore, NAC supports other antioxidants, including vitamins C and E and glutathione, and fights free-radical damage that impairs mental functions, too. Because it is a potent detoxifying agent, NAC is often used to treat acetaminophen (Tylenol) poisoning, and it may be useful in reducing cellular damage from environmental pollutants.

DOSAGE: A typical dosage of NAC is 250 to 500 mg, one to three times daily for both women and men.

FOODS: NAC is not found in food.

Quercetin

A member of the group of compounds known as flavonoids, quercetin has repeatedly demonstrated strong antioxidant capabilities, making it a useful weapon in fighting the free-radical damage that harms hearing. It is actively being studied as a remedy for a number of different conditions, including allergies, cancer, inflammation, and cardiovascular disease. The heart, for example, gets a boost from quercetin's ability to reduce the formation of LDL ("bad") cholesterol and to keep blood vessels strong and flexible. In addition, quercetin may help reduce high blood pressure and strengthen blood vessels.

DOSAGE: Up to 400 mg per day for both women and men is considered safe.

FOODS: Quercetin is found in a wide variety of fruits and vegetables, including onions, apples, kale, green tea, red cabbage, tomatoes, green beans, lettuce, grapes, and potatoes.

Resveratrol

A compound found in red wine, grapes, and grape juice, resveratrol is shaping up as a key player in the Save Your Hearing Now Program. Research conducted by my colleagues and I found that resveratrol provided significant protection for the ears during exposure to loud noises.[21] Other studies have found that resveratrol extends life spans in yeast by as much as 80 percent, putting it on a par with serious calorie restriction for slowing the aging process. It also may ward off neurodegenerative diseases, like Alzheimer's and Parkinson's, and protect the heart by reducing LDL ("bad") cholesterol levels.[22]

DOSAGE: A daily dose of 25 to 100 mg for both women and men is typical.

FOODS: Red wine, red grapes and grape juice, mulberries, and peanuts all contain resveratrol.

Zinc

Like many other minerals, zinc is involved in hundreds of processes in the body. For example, it assists in metabolism, insulin production, and the manufacture of RNA and DNA, which enables cells to repair, grow, and divide. Zinc has potent antioxidant abilities, which not only counteract free radicals but also make it useful for reducing the effects of aging. Zinc also increases the effectiveness of other antioxidants. For example, it manages levels of vitamin E in the blood and enhances vitamin A absorption. Since the highest levels of zinc in the body are found in the inner ear and eye, it is essential for good hearing.

Recently, zinc's immune-enhancing properties have been tested as a remedy for the common cold, with promising results. Zinc is actually one of the elements that make up superoxide dismutase (SOD), one of the antioxidants produced in the body, although production typically declines with age.

Individuals with low levels of zinc might experience immune problems, such as repeated infections or wounds that are slow to heal, as well as acne, prostate difficulties, impotence, or diminished ability to taste or smell.

Birth control pills, diuretics, some types of antibiotics, diabetes, liver and kidney diseases, a high-fiber diet, and even excessive sweating can reduce levels of zinc in the body.

DOSAGE: The RDA is 12 mg for women and 15 mg for men. Doses of 25 to 100 mg per day are considered safe, but higher levels can backfire, causing problems for the immune system. *Caution:* Zinc should not be taken at the same time as iron, since these two minerals cancel one another's benefits. Furthermore, zinc intake needs to be balanced with the mineral copper, since taking high levels of zinc can deplete copper supplies, and vice versa. The appropriate ratio of copper to zinc is 1:10.

FOODS: Brewer's yeast, liver, egg yolks, lima beans, mushrooms, seafood (oysters in particular), and whole grains contain zinc.

HOW TO BUY AND USE SUPPLEMENTS

1. First, the cautions: If you are pregnant, nursing, have diabetes, are currently taking prescription medication, or are under a doctor's care for a chronic health condition, consult a health care expert with advanced nutrition training, such as a holistic nutritionist.

2. The best nutritional supplements are those that typically exceed the recommended daily allowances. Thus, the common one-a-day supplements are not the best choice. (In the Resources section, we offer some suggestions.) Check labels and look for "all-natural" ingredients, which are better absorbed. Also pay close attention to the serving size noted on the label. The "Supplement Facts" label lists the total amount of each nutrient the multivitamin provides *per serving*, not per pill. In some cases, this level is only obtained by taking more than one pill. If a nutrient amount is listed in micrograms (mcg), the product supplies very little of it. In some cases, such as certain B vitamins, mcg are appropriate, but with other nutrients, such as CoQ10, they are not. Some vitamin companies have misleading statements on their labels, suggesting that they

contain high levels of specific nutrients. The only way to tell if they actually do is to read the fine print.

3. Many people ask if there isn't just one pill they can take and get on with their lives. The answer is no. To take advantage of the Save Your Hearing Now Program, you will have to take ten or more pills throughout the day.

4. When purchasing a mineral supplement, look for a product that has been chelated with amino acids, as this process significantly enhances the absorption. This is especially true for anyone over the age of thirty-five, because the gastrointestinal tract absorbs only about 2 to 12 percent of all minerals. Chelation increases the absorption rate to 40 percent or more.

5. Pay attention to the label's fine print, which tells whether or not the nutrients are in natural form. Natural vitamin E (shown as d-alphatocopherol on the label), for example, is far more useful for the body than the synthetic (dl-alphatocopherol). A product that also includes the form of vitamin E known as mixed tocopherols is an excellent choice, even though it may cost more.

6. Unless package directions state otherwise, always take supplements with a little food or a meal and eight ounces of water.

7. If you're new to the world of supplements, you may be surprised to find that product labels offer very little information in terms of what conditions a nutrient might be good for. That's because the Dietary Supplement Health and Education Act of 1994 (DSHEA) oversees claims and provides labeling requirements to give consumers a reasonable degree of safety. DSHEA allows the federal government to remove products from the market that may endanger health.

Beyond the Basics

Now that you have been introduced to the Top Ten nutrients of the Save Your Hearing Now Program, let's go beyond the basics and look at other substances that support those compounds while providing additional support for good hearing. Although these compounds may not necessarily have a direct link to protecting the auditory system, they are important for other reasons. For example, as I noted earlier, a healthy cardiovascular system and adequate circulation are essential for good hearing. As a result, many of these supplements are recommended for their role in heart and circulatory health because both benefit the auditory system. Here are some other nutrients that play an important role in the Save Your Hearing Now Program:

The Top Ten's Supporting Players

Many of these nutrients are found in multivitamin/mineral formulas, so they are not difficult to obtain.

vitamin A	copper
beta-carotene	magnesium
vitamin C	manganese
vitamin D	molybdenum
vitamin E	potassium
boron	selenium
calcium	green tea extract

Vitamin A

A potent antioxidant and essential nutrient, vitamin A is involved in a wide range of bodily operations, from vision and reproduction to cell division and differentiation, the process by which a cell determines what it is going to become. Vitamin A also supports health of the immune system.

Preliminary studies are showing that vitamin A may play a role in hearing, too. An award-winning study from Belgium, for example, demonstrated that vitamin A was effective in regenerating and repairing inner ear hair cells.[23]

DOSAGE: The current RDA for vitamin A is 4,000 IU for a healthy adult woman and 5,000 IU for a man. *Caution:* Megadoses of this nutrient can be toxic and have also been linked to bone fractures in men and women, so stay within recommended limits unless a physician recommends and supervises larger amounts.

FOODS: Green and yellow vegetables, as well as liver, are good sources of vitamin A.

Beta-Carotene

Beta-carotene is a member of the carotenoid family, a group of plant pigments with outstanding health benefits that are only beginning to be studied. Several carotenoids have the ability to convert to vitamin A in the digestive tract, and beta-carotene is one of them. Beta-carotene's antioxidant capabilities make it useful for protecting hearing. The added bonus of beta-carotene is that it does not accumulate in the body, so there is no danger of overdose, as there is with vitamin A.

DOSAGE: There is no established RDA for beta-carotene. However, dosages between 6 and 30 mg (the equivalent of 5,000 to 25,000 IU) per day for both women and men are considered safe. Smokers, however, should not take more than 2,500 to 5,000 IU per day of beta-carotene. At least two studies have demonstrated an increased risk of lung cancer among those who smoke and take more than 5,000 IU of beta-carotene.

FOODS: Beta-carotene is one of the most common carotenoids in fruits and vegetables. It is the orange color found in carrots, pumpkins, peaches, sweet potatoes, and other similarly colored foods.

Vitamin C

Although it has a reputation as a cold fighter, there is an impressive body of research showing that vitamin C can do much more than help fight sniffles. A hardworking antioxidant, vitamin C offers two added bonuses: It helps the body deal with stress, and it boosts vitamin E activity, making it a good antiaging choice. There is also a definite hearing link: New research with lab animals shows that consuming levels of the nutrient higher than those found in the typical diet can protect against noise-induced hearing loss.[24]

Although other mammals can produce vitamin C in the body, humans cannot. Studies have shown that Americans tend to consume far too few vitamin C–rich foods. Doses of vitamin C found in most multivitamins tend to be low, so additional supplements are recommended. Since it is water-soluble, excess C is flushed from the body in the urine, so there is not much danger of overdosing. Ideally, vitamin C supplements should be taken several times a day, to maintain sufficient levels in the body.

DOSAGE: The RDA is 75 mg for women and 90 mg for men. As part of the Save Your Hearing Now Program, however, I recommend taking a total of anywhere from 100 to 1,500 mg daily, in divided doses. As much as 2,000 mg per day is considered safe. Linus Pauling, a famous Nobel laureate, advocated 10,000 mg per day, an amount that is probably too high for the average person.

FOODS: Fresh fruits, especially citrus, cantaloupe, berries, and mango, and many vegetables contain vitamin C.

Vitamin D

After being ignored for years, a number of new studies have put vitamin D in the limelight. Or maybe we should say in the "sunlight," since vitamin D is often called the sunshine vitamin. Our bodies can produce this nutrient with small amounts of sun exposure (fifteen minutes, three times a week) on bare skin without sunscreen. Yes, that goes contrary to all the warnings about sun exposure and skin cancer. But vitamin D's supporters, a group that includes some high-profile scientists, insist this small amount of sun is safe and may even reduce the risk of certain cancers.

Supplements are inexpensive, and the benefits are turning out to be significant, from building strong bones and fighting depression to avoiding cancer. Interestingly, in the mid-1980s, hearing loss was linked to a deficiency of vitamin D by a German researcher who found that hearing could often be restored by giving the patient vitamin D supplements.[25]

DOSAGE: Recommendations for daily intake of vitamin D have recently been revised. Instead of an RDA, the federal government now recommends that adult men and women up to age fifty take 200 IU per day. Between ages fifty-one and seventy, the AI is 400 IU daily, and after seventy-one it is 600 IU. Since vitamin D is fat-soluble and therefore can accumulate in the body, megadoses (more than 65,000 IU daily) are not recommended.

FOODS: Many dairy products are fortified with vitamin D, and the nutrient is also found in eggs, fish liver oils, and some fatty types of fish.

Vitamin E

Another superstar antioxidant, vitamin E is closely linked to heart health and enhanced circulation, both of which support the auditory system. At the cellular level, vitamin E is essential for healthy membranes. It can be challenging to get sufficient vitamin E from diet alone, because this fat-soluble nutrient is found in fairly small amounts in food, and cooking and processing eliminate much of it. One expert estimated that achieving levels of vitamin E that could lower the risk of cardiovascular disease would require eating nine tablespoons of olive oil, seventy-five slices of whole-wheat bread, and forty almonds or two hundred peanuts each and every day.

DOSAGE: The RDA is 8 mg for women and 10 mg for men, which is the equivalent of 12 to 15 IU per day. Typically, supplements containing 200 to 800 IU or more are considered safe. Some clinical trials have demonstrated that 800 to 1,200 IU may be required to affect cardiovascular health, particularly in patients who already have heart disease, so those with heart disease should consult a physician. Natural vitamin E, labeled as d-alphatocopherol, is the most bioavailable form. *Caution:* Individuals who are taking blood-thinning medications should discuss appropriate doses of vitamin E with a physician, since the combination of large doses of vitamin E and these drugs may result in bleeding and delayed clotting.

FOODS: Nuts, olive oil, whole-grain bread, soybeans, and some seeds supply small amounts of vitamin E.

THE TRUTH ABOUT THE VITAMIN E CONTROVERSY

If you caught any of the media reports on the dangers of vitamin E, you may be wondering about the safety of these supplements. The good news is there's no reason to worry. Although several stories made it sound as though vitamin E was dangerous, those conclusions are misinterpretations of what a particular study actually found. The dire warnings were based on a meta-analysis by researchers at Johns Hopkins. The scientists reviewed nineteen previously published articles, involving roughly 136,000 patients, and determined that consuming more than 400 IU of vitamin E per day may increase the risk of dying by 6 percent.[26]

Not surprisingly, the media trumpeted the bad-news aspect of the story, without providing any details. And, as is so often the case with scientific findings, "sound bites" simply can't tell the whole story. The first thing vitamin E's defenders point to is the fact that the research had shortcomings. The studies that were reviewed, for example, consisted largely of older individuals who were already suffering chronic illness of one sort or another, including Alzheimer's, Parkinson's, and kidney failure, as well as a group of smokers. It's difficult to imagine that vitamin E alone could improve the health of these individuals.

Second, while some of the studies focused on vitamin E exclusively, a number of others included a variety of vitamins, including E. From a statistical standpoint, mixing such a wide assortment of studies together can produce meaningless results. Third, they eliminated twelve studies that showed a low likelihood of dying, creating a very serious bias against a positive outcome. Finally, it should be noted that the Johns Hopkins researchers themselves pointed out that because most of the patients in these trials had chronic illness and were over the age of sixty, the study's findings might not necessarily apply to younger, healthy individuals.

If the media had told the whole story about vitamin E, reporters would have mentioned numerous studies showing that an increased intake of antioxidants, such as vitamin E, reduces the incidence of heart disease, stroke, Alzheimer's disease, and cancer. In addition, vitamin E has also been shown to boost immune function and to combat free-radical damage. As you can see, when it comes to health and supplements in the news, it pays to get the whole story.

The Mighty Minerals and More

Moving right along, let's take some of the mystery out of minerals, especially the lesser known, "trace" minerals. Our bodies only need very small amounts of these substances, but that doesn't mean they are insignificant. Here are the trace minerals and other substances that are recommended to support the Save Your Hearing Now Top Ten:

Boron

Boron is involved in both bone and brain health and assists in magnesium, calcium, and vitamin D metabolism. Because vitamin D deficiencies can affect hearing, boron is indirectly involved in protecting hearing.

DOSAGE: There is no established RDA or AI for boron, but doses of 3 mg daily are considered safe.

FOODS: Leafy vegetables, apples, avocado, carrots, dried beans, grape juice, peanuts and peanut butter, pecans, prune juice, and wine contain boron.

Calcium

Renowned for its connection to strong bones, calcium is actually essential for many bodily functions, from the nervous system to cell wall strength and flexibility. There is no direct link to hearing, but since calcium is involved in maintaining a healthy cardiovascular system, it should not be overlooked. It also assists in metabolizing vitamin B_{12}, which does have a direct link to the auditory system.

DOSAGE: 1,000 to 1,200 mg per day is the average adult dosage, but 1,500 mg daily is often recommended for postmenopausal women and men at risk for osteoporosis.

FOODS: Dairy products, salmon, sardines, kale, broccoli, nuts, beans, tofu, and chickpeas are all good sources of calcium.

Copper

Copper must be balanced with zinc and vitamin C intake and works with those two nutrients to keep the skin healthy, among other things. Its role in protecting hearing comes from its connection to the antioxidant enzyme superoxide dismutase (SOD), which fights aging by reducing free-radical damage.

DOSAGE: The RDA is 900 mcg for both women and men, but 2 mg is a more typical dose.

FOODS: Avocado, oysters, organ meats, beets, salmon, wholegrain bread and cereal, dark green leafy vegetables, dried legumes, nuts, soybeans, and chocolate.

Magnesium

Magnesium has repeatedly been proven to be effective at combating noise-induced hearing loss, in animal studies and in research with military recruits who were exposed to high levels of noise during basic training.[27] In addition, magnesium is important because literally hundreds of enzyme processes depend on it. For example, it is essential for a healthy heart and good circulation, as well as managing blood pressure. Once abundant in the farmland of this country, the mineral is now in short supply, so food may not be the best source. According to a report by the USDA, three-quarters of the American population consumes inadequate amounts of magnesium.

DOSAGE: The RDA is 310 mg for women and 400 mg for men.

FOODS: Brewer's yeast, dairy products, brown rice, dark green leafy vegetables, legumes, whole grains, and nuts are sources of magnesium.

Manganese

Without manganese, our bodies would have difficulty producing a number of enzymes that are necessary for metabolizing cholesterol, protein, and amino acids. Manganese plays a role in bone health and is also required to produce one of the body's most effective antioxidants, superoxide dismutase (SOD), so this mineral has an antiaging connection.

DOSAGE: There is no RDA, but the AI levels are 1.8 mg per day for women and 2.3 mg for men.

FOODS: Nuts, avocado, seaweed, whole-grain bread and cereal, dried beans and peas, and pineapple are sources of manganese.

Molybdenum

One of the unsung heroes of the mineral world, molybdenum is involved in essential cellular functions and plays a role in keeping the liver, the body's leading detoxification organ, healthy. We only need a very small amount of this nutrient. Deficiencies have been linked to cancer.

DOSAGE: The RDA is 45 mcg for both women and men. Up to 500 mcg per day is considered safe.

FOODS: Dark green leafy vegetables, legumes, beans, and peas contain molybdenum.

Potassium

Potassium is involved in everything from heart health to transporting nutrients into and out of cells. It also plays a role in maintaining healthy blood pressure levels and promotes good circulation, especially in later years. Potassium has no known direct link to hearing, but it clearly supports the work of the Top Ten.

DOSAGE: There is no RDA, but the AI levels are 4.7 grams per day for both women and men. Since potassium is fairly easy to obtain from food, supplements of 100 mg or less are typical.

FOODS: Potatoes, bananas, dairy products, meat, peanuts, brown rice, and brewer's yeast are a few good sources.

Selenium

A key antioxidant, selenium is vitally important in a number of processes within the body and has been linked to cardiovascular health, as well as enhanced immunity and protection against various types of cancer. Selenium works especially well with vitamin E, because these two antioxidants enhance each other's absorption.

DOSAGE: The RDA is 55 mcg for both women and men. All selenium is not created equal, though. Personally, I recommend selenium that comes from a yeast source or selenium methionate.

FOODS: Brazil nuts, brewer's yeast, brown rice, molasses, salmon, and whole grains are sources of selenium.

Green Tea Extract

For centuries, green tea has been the beverage of choice in Asia, where it is renowned for its therapeutic properties. Science is now confirming that green tea does indeed offer health benefits, including fighting cancer and lowering cholesterol. It contains several highly regarded antioxidants, including EGCG (epigallocatechin gallate), which is currently the focus of a number of studies. These beneficial antioxidants make it useful for protecting the auditory system.

DOSAGE: There is no RDA for green tea. In capsule form, a typical dose is 500 mg of a standardized extract. If you enjoy it as a beverage, four or five cups of green tea is recommended. (See also page 130 for more about the health benefits of green tea.)

Supplements are the foundation of the Save Your Hearing Now Program because there is considerable evidence that various substances protect against the mitochondrial damage that causes hearing loss and aging. Of course, the supplements need support from a varied, nutritious diet, the second step in the program. In the next chapter, we will take a look at how easy it is to make the dietary changes that support the Save Your Hearing Now Program.

((**7**))

STEP TWO: A SOUND DIET STRATEGY

"Leave your drugs in the chemist's pot if you can heal the patient with food." —HIPPOCRATES

Katherine's years of coaching women's high school basketball and being part of an active bowling league had led to hearing loss that finally caught up with her in her late forties. She was no longer able to hear conversations during meetings at the high school where she worked, and she was wondering if there was anything she could do to change that, short of investing in hearing aids.

Fortunately, Katherine was interested in alternative remedies and was already taking some supplements, so she was more than happy to follow my recommendations. But she was intrigued by the fact that I had a background in nutrition, and asked if there was any remedy for the "middle-age spread" she was experiencing. So we spent some time discussing food.

Katherine, like so many people facing weight issues, had tried one diet after another. She would lose weight and then regain it. Frustration was getting the best of her, so she began skipping breakfast and lunch. But the weight still didn't budge. "When I was younger, if I missed even one meal, I'd be a couple pounds lighter the next day. Now it doesn't matter if I starve myself all day. I'm thinking about having liposuction, just so I can button my skirts and pants again."

I explained to Katherine how the very things she was doing were contributing to her weight problem. Based on our talk, and Katherine's own research, she turned over a new dietary leaf. In essence, Katherine gave up dieting, meal skipping, and the microwave approach to cooking, which involved a great deal of frozen, ready-made "meals." Instead, she focused on what she called a cleansing diet, centered on organic, whole foods, especially fruits and vegetables, grains, and lean protein. She also joined a neighborhood group that walked two miles every evening after work.

After about ten days, Katherine started noticing that things were changing for the better. She felt less moody, had more energy, and slept through the night. And even though it was challenging to live without the convenience foods, Katherine felt it was well worth it. I saw her again at three months, and she reported even more improvements. She was especially gratified when several people at work, who noticed how much better she was doing, decided to follow her example. At six months, Katherine called to tell me that she thought she was losing her mind. Her hearing, which had definitely been failing, seemed to have stabilized. Since she was not the first person to report this, I assured her that she should not be concerned about her sanity—her hearing loss was indeed repaired, at least in part, by the supplements and lifestyle changes, including her new, vastly improved diet.

How Food Became a Four-Letter Word

As you have no doubt heard, America is currently in the grip of an obesity epidemic. More than 60 percent of the adults in the United States are considered overweight or obese, and more children than ever before are carrying extra pounds, too. Weight is not just a cosmetic concern. Statistics reported in a recent issue of the journal *Health Affairs* stated that the extra costs to private insurance related to caring for the obese soared from 2 percent of the total in 1987 to 11.6 percent in 2002.[1] The report did not include costs to Medicare and Medicaid, but there is little doubt that excess-weight-related health care expenses are driving up the cost of these tax-financed programs as well. Ironically, in the midst of it all, Americans are spending more than $40 billion on diet and weight loss products each year!

Not only are weight-related health care costs in the United States soaring, but experts say obesity-related ailments are well on the way to becoming a leading cause of death. The combination of processed and junk foods with a sedentary lifestyle is now considered lethal; some 300,000 deaths are attributed to it each year, according to a 2001 study by the Office of the Surgeon General.

Excess weight has been linked to a variety of health concerns, including heart disease, high blood pressure, diabetes, certain types of cancer, arthritis, and more. The health problems associated with extra pounds were clearly defined by a study conducted at the Fred Hutchinson Cancer Research Center in Seattle with more than 73,000 middle-aged adults. Researchers looked at the incidence of forty-one common health concerns, including seven serious diseases and two conditions linked to heart disease, and then tried to determine if excess weight increased the likelihood of being diagnosed with these chronic ailments. They found that for women, thirty-seven of the forty-one conditions were associated with an increase in BMI (body mass index, a measure of height to weight ratio), while twenty-nine of the forty-one had a similar connection for men.[2]

How Weight Harms Hearing

How is obesity or excess weight related to hearing? Although that subject is only beginning to be studied, Swedish researchers did find a connection recently. They followed nearly three hundred Swedish women over a twenty-four-year period. Using various data, including physical exams and brain scans, they found the first evidence that those with a high BMI throughout adult life had lost brain tissue when compared to women with lower BMIs. Loss of brain tissue occurred in the temporal lobe portion of the brain, where the auditory system is located, along with language, speech, memory, and comprehension.[3]

Why would weight affect the brain? There are three possible answers to that question. One, excess weight could increase the number of damaging free radicals in the body. Two, fat may produce harmful substances, such as growth factors and hormones, which can erode brain tissue. And three, excess fat might be responsible for hardening of the arteries (atherosclerosis) and result in limited oxygen flow to the brain.

Another connection between obesity and hearing loss is suggested by recent findings from Great Britain linking excess weight with accelerated aging. In a study involving more than eleven hundred women, scientists found that obesity had a greater effect on markers of aging than smoking. Among women who were obese, the markers showed signs of aging that were the equivalent of nearly nine years beyond those who were lean. Not surprisingly, being overweight or obese increases free-radical levels in the body, which the experts believe to be the reason more signs of aging were seen in those of excess weight.[4]

Defining "Healthy" Weight

Maintaining a "healthy" weight means keeping your BMI at a reasonable level. You can figure out where you fall on a BMI chart with pencil and paper, or a calculator, or by visiting the National Heart, Lung, and Blood Institute's Web page at http://nhlbisupport.com/bmi/bmicalc.htm or the Centers for Disease Control version at http://www.cdc.gov/nccdphp/dnpa/bmi/calc-bmi.htm. You can also calculate your BMI at my Web site by going to http://www.bodylanguagevitamin.com and clicking on Educational Resources on the task bar at the left.

For those who are comfortable with a little math, here is the do-it-yourself method. Let's say an individual is five feet five inches tall and weighs 156 pounds. First, convert height to inches and square it (i.e., multiply it times itself). Five feet five inches tall is the same as sixty-five inches, and multiplying 65 times 65 produces 4,225. Now divide 4,225 into the number of pounds (156). The result is 0.036. Now multiply 0.036 by 703. The resulting figure, 25.3, indicates that this individual is a bit overweight.

BMI Categories

Underweight	Below 18.5
Normal weight	Between 18.6 and 24.9
Overweight	Between 25 and 29.9
Obese	30 or more

Although the BMI is considered an accurate means of determining an appropriate weight for an individual's height, it is not foolproof. Serious athletes and bodybuilders may fall into overweight or obese categories simply because muscle weighs more than fat. On the other hand, individuals at the opposite end of the spectrum who have little muscle mass may score in the normal range, even though they are overweight. But by and large, the BMI is a useful tool for most people to determine whether or not they are at a healthy weight. I would like to emphasize, however, that even slender and healthy-weight individuals can benefit from the Save Your Hearing Now nutrition advice. The purpose here is not weight loss per se, but an increase in antioxidants and other nutrients that support health throughout the body, with a special focus on the ears.

Better Food Equals Better Hearing

Lifestyle plays an enormous role in obesity, heart disease, diabetes, arthritis, and a host of other conditions that can affect our hearing. Food choices make up a significant part of lifestyle. Many people are looking for advice on how to make healthful food choices, and who can blame them? Experts don't agree, one study contradicts the next, and fad diets come and go at a head-spinning pace. At some point, people become frustrated and decide to eat whatever is handy and tastes good. Unfortunately, that approach is a recipe for disaster, affecting both health and hearing. So let's look at some simple ways to improve the average diet that are quick and easy, as well as healthful.

If you're interested in losing weight but are wondering why you can't just eat a little less of your normal fare and not make so many changes, a few points should be noted. If a "normal" meal to you is fast food or something processed or prepared, you're most likely getting bombarded with sodium, sugar, unhealthful fats, and very little in the way of nutrition.

This type of food satisfies the taste buds and may fill your stomach, but it accomplishes little in terms of promoting good health.

Here is why. Fast and prepared foods are notoriously high in calories and low in nutrients. Eating empty calories leaves the body hungry for more. One of the paradoxes of our time is that Americans are increasingly overweight and yet malnourished at the same time. Following the food guidelines in the Save Your Hearing Now Program does require making some changes, but you will be providing your body with the nutrients it needs to function at its best.

The next section begins with a brief overview of the four basic elements of the Save Your Hearing Now Program's nutrition advice. Then we summarize relevant nutrition research to explain why these four elements are important, and explain the simple steps you can take to put this advice to work for you. Finally, in the section titled "How to Eat," you'll find additional research-based pointers that provide further support for healthy hearing.

As in Chapter Six, where we considered a large number of supplements and noted how each was connected to hearing, here we explain how specific foods and eating habits play a role in the Save Your Hearing Now Program. Let's get started.

The Save Your Hearing Now Food Program

Whether you want to simply protect your hearing, lose weight, or just feed your body well, eating nutritious food is the place to start. The four steps that follow are based on solid science and respected research. They are designed to make dietary improvements as simple and effective as possible.

1. Focus on whole foods with high antioxidant and fiber content.
2. Get to know the "good" fats and increase your intake of them.
3. Reduce intake of refined and processed ingredients, especially sugar and high-fructose corn syrup.
4. Do not diet, but do practice moderation when food and drink are involved.

Now let's look at why these four guidelines are the foundation of the program and how to incorporate them into daily life.

Whole Foods Provide Antioxidants and More

What exactly are whole foods? Essentially, these are the non-processed, unrefined foods that were commonplace in our diet before white bread, sodas, and packaged, convenience foods were invented. Fruits and vegetables are whole foods, for example, as are whole grains.

Whole foods are first on the list because they are abundant sources of antioxidants, so they support the supplements that can protect hearing. The most powerful food sources of these all-important nutrients are vegetables and fruits, so they should be included in each and every meal and snack. If you are accustomed to eating prepared, processed, or fast foods, whole foods may seem like a gigantic leap into the unknown. Often, when I mention this sort of dietary change to patients, they start to explain all the reasons why they can't possibly manage to do this—no time, too complicated, they hate "bird food," and so on. I have to agree that for many people, improving eating habits is a challenge. But the bottom line is this: Making these changes can have far-reaching health benefits, including a longer, healthier life, which means more quality time with family and friends.

There is plenty of proof of just how powerful a diet like this can be to good health. One study published in the *New England Journal of Medicine*, for example, examined the eating habits of more than 22,000 men and women in Greece for four years. Those whose meals were most focused on vegetables, fruits, whole grains, fish and poultry and good fats like olive oil—in other words, the Mediterranean diet—had a lower risk of dying from both heart disease and stroke, two leading killers in many countries, including our own.[5]

All fruits and vegetables are not created equal, however. The ORAC (Oxygen Radical Absorbance Capacity) analysis is a good yardstick for determining which fruits and vegetables to put at the top of the shopping list. Scientists at the USDA have developed this rating scale to measure the antioxidant content of various plant foods. The foods at the top of the ORAC scale contain as much as twenty times the antioxidant power of other foods. When researchers compared lab animals who were supplied with foods high on the ORAC list with those on a low-ORAC diet, they found that members of the first group were biologically younger in areas such as ability to balance, strength of the tiny blood vessels known as capillaries, and brain functions such as memory.

ORAC Superstars

FRUITS	ORAC Units in 3.5 Ounces
Prunes	5,770
Raisins	2,830
Blueberries	2,400

FRUITS	ORAC Units in 3.5 Ounces
Blackberries	2,036
Strawberries	1,540
Raspberries	1,220
Plums	949
Oranges	750
Red grapes	739

VEGETABLES	ORAC Units in 3.5 Ounces
Kale	1,770
Spinach	1,260
Brussels sprouts	980
Alfalfa sprouts	930
Broccoli florets	890
Beets	840
Red bell peppers	710
Onions	450
Corn	400

From the USDA Web site.

A reasonable goal is to consume about 3,000 ORAC units a day. If you sprinkle half a cup of blueberries (2,400 units) on breakfast cereal or have a spinach salad (1,260) and snack on an orange (750) and some red grapes (739), you're home free. Let's go a step farther though, because the ORAC scale is not the whole story.

Beyond ORAC

To really ramp up antioxidant intake from whole foods, start sampling from a wide variety of differently colored fruits and vegetables. Why? Because these foods are filled with assorted phytochemicals—known as carotenoids and flavonoids—that have been shown to provide tremendous health benefits.

Basically, carotenoids are pigments, the substances that make carrots orange, corn yellow, and tomatoes red. Many flavonoids are pigments, too, although some provide flavor, as their name suggests. Carotenoids and flavonoids also have significant antioxidant properties and support the work of other antioxidants.

Research has shown that carotenoids can help protect the body from heart disease, cancer, diabetes, Alzheimer's disease, chronic fatigue syndrome, and vision problems. Better-known carotenoids, such as beta-carotene, lutein, and lycopene, have been researched extensively. Scientists now know that some of them are able to convert to other nutrients as the body needs them, while others target certain diseases. Beta-carotene, the precursor to vitamin A, for example, boosts activity of the immune cells to shield us against infections and some forms of cancer. The risk of macular degeneration, a leading cause of blindness, decreases with lutein, while studies focusing on lycopene have shown that this carotenoid can protect against prostate, stomach, and lung cancers.

Carotenoids' cousins, the flavonoids, are substances found not only in fruits and vegetables but in tea, nuts, beans, herbs, legumes, and grains. Of the thousands of flavonoids in existence, some have been studied, including genistein, a soybean derivative, and green tea's EGCG (epigallocatechin gallate). Both have demonstrated impressive health benefits, ranging from supporting heart health to fighting cancer.

Carotenoids and flavonoids are only the tip of the iceberg,

though, when it comes to the power of whole foods. Two quick examples: Ellagic acid, a substance related to carotenoids and flavonoids, has been the subject of studies examining its cancer-fighting capabilities. The results show that ellagic acid slows the growth of cancer cells. Meanwhile, a compound known as perillyl alcohol (just a chemical term, not really intoxicating), found in tart cherries, is another outstanding cancer-fighter.

ARE ORGANIC FOODS REALLY BETTER?

Although the subject is still controversial, a growing body of research shows that organic produce has greater health-promoting properties than nonorganic produce. For example, research has found that organic fruits and vegetables contain higher levels of vitamin C, as well as polyphenols, the umbrella term for the carotenoid/flavonoid family (and other nutrient groups).

It makes sense that organic produce would contain more carotenoids and flavonoids, because the original purpose of these substances was to protect plants from pests and other dangers. Since they are not treated with pesticides, organically grown fruits and vegetables must manufacture their own form of protection with greater amounts of carotenoids, flavonoids, and related compounds. Logically, that translates into higher levels of these substances for those of us who eat them.

Furthermore, eating organic produce means fewer harmful synthetic pesticides in the body. A recent study conducted by scientists at the University of Washington, Emory University, and the Centers for Disease Control and Prevention found that when children eat organic foods, the level of pesticides in their bodies falls dramatically and immediately.[6]

Conventionally grown foods with the highest levels of

pesticide residues are peaches, apples, pears, grapes, green beans, spinach, winter squash, strawberries, and cantaloupe. The lowest levels of pesticides in conventionally grown foods are found in bananas, broccoli, canned peaches, canned or frozen peas, canned or frozen corn, milk, orange juice, apple juice, and grape juice. Pesticide residue levels can be reduced by washing and peeling produce whenever possible.

Remember, too, that fruits and vegetables are not the only food sources of pesticides. Conventionally grown grains are also treated with these substances, but organic bread, cereal, rice, and pasta are widely available.

Whole foods are excellent sources of carotenoids, flavonoids, and no doubt other substances that have not yet been recognized. Many of these compounds are only beginning to be researched, so their link to good hearing is not known. But, as we have seen, antioxidants in general support good hearing by protecting against free-radical damage, so logic tells us that the compounds in whole foods are likely to be beneficial. Moreover, there is really no downside to eating a diet rich in fruits, vegetables, whole grains, legumes, and nuts. Whole foods are not expensive, they taste great (although, admittedly, this type of eating plan may take some getting used to, especially if you're accustomed to junk and fast foods), and they are good for us.

In addition to providing your body with the building blocks of good health, there's one more area where whole foods excel—weight management. A diet rich in these foods falls into the high-carbohydrate, high-fiber category. In addition, the carbohydrates in these foods are primarily complex, the very kind that provide the slow, steady supply of energy essential for managing hunger and preventing cravings from undermining weight loss efforts.

Although the Standard American Diet is not built around these foods, we can start changing that by trading in processed and prepared goods, fast food, and snacks for "real" food—fruits, vegetables, grains, and nuts.

Quick Tips

Choose organic food over conventionally grown. Organic produce usually costs a little more, but the pesticides and herbicides used in conventionally grown foods have been linked to weight gain.

Choose food before supplements. Most nutritionists agree that there are very likely beneficial substances in whole foods that have not yet been identified. So, yes, you can get vitamin C from a supplement rather than from an orange, but the orange is loaded with other things your body needs, including antioxidants, fiber, and very likely healthful substances that haven't even been discovered yet! For nutrient information on hundreds of foods, visit the USDA's Nutrient Data Laboratory at http://www.nal.usda.gov/fnic/foodcomp.

Drink Your Way to Better Nutrition

Americans love their coffee, but it's hard to ignore the tremendous benefits of drinking tea. Loaded with healthful compounds known as polyphenols, tea is hard to beat when it comes to beverages that benefit health.

Scientists have been focusing on several specific tea substances, including amino acid L-theanine and the polyphenol EGCG (epigallocatechin gallate). While EGCG appears to have significant anticancer properties, L-theanine, found in both black and green teas, has been linked to better heart and brain health. Japanese researchers, for example, found that L-theanine in green tea protected animal brain cells from damage and death by preventing the formation of LDL ("bad") cholesterol. Another study, also from Japan, tested forty-three different tea polyphenols to determine if their antioxidant ability could inhibit the development of LDL cholesterol. All but three performed better than vitamin E.[7] Reducing cholesterol and maintaining a healthy heart is recommended for good hearing.

If you are still not convinced that it's time to turn off the coffeepot, consider this: Tea is turning out to be helpful in weight loss. A Swiss study demonstrated that a combination of green tea extract and caffeine stimulated an additional 3 to 4 percent weight loss in men as compared with those who were given only caffeine or a placebo.[8] Furthermore, USDA researchers supported those findings when they compared calorie-burning among men who drank five cups of black (oolong) tea daily with those who drank plain water and another group consuming caffeinated water. Those in the caffeinated water group scored highest—3.4 percent more calorie expenditure than the water drinkers—but black tea was a close second with 2.9 percent more calories burned.[9]

Right now the experts believe that drinking four or five cups of green or black tea daily produces health benefits. Green tea extract in supplement form is another option, but some nutritionists believe the real thing is better.

If you've tried green tea and don't like the way it tastes, here are a couple of suggestions. First, try it again. All kinds of new versions are now available, designed to appeal to the American palate, with fruit and other flavors reducing the bitterness. Also try white tea and rooibos (*roy*-boss), or red, tea.

White tea is less processed than either green or black tea, and it contains higher levels of antioxidants. Low in caffeine, white tea produces very little color, and the taste is very mild. The powerhouse antioxidant EGCG is more abundant in white tea than in green or black tea. EGCG provides protection against cancer and promotes good heart health.

Although it is not technically a tea because it is derived from a bush, rooibos is a South African favorite that's caffeine-free, contains plenty of antioxidants, and has a distinctive robust flavor that goes very well with milk or cream. Studies from around the world show that the antioxidants in rooibos tea offer a long list of health and antiaging benefits.

If you are like me and never learned to drink teas or coffees, you can take organically grown green tea leaves, crush them, and swallow them. Yes, they taste terrible, but it is another way to get the "medicine" they contain. A tastier option is to take a look at several books available on cooking with teas. In this case, different types of tea are used as seasonings, and the results can be truly outstanding.

Fiber: The Unsung Hero of Health

Fiber is another reason to eat more whole foods. The Standard American Diet is virtually fiber-free, and that's not good. Fiber is loaded with health-enhancing nutrients. And, because it consists of complex carbohydrates, it is digested more slowly than refined-grain foods, like white bread, white rice, and many popular cereals. Eating fiber-rich foods can help with weight loss, too. A bowl of all-bran or steel-cut oatmeal (sorry, not the instant variety) provides a steady source of fuel and wards off hunger pangs for much longer than a doughnut does.

With so much attention devoted to fat these days, fiber's role in good health is getting shortchanged, and that's a shame. Fiber is a real health hero. In fact, because it contains impressive nutrients and encourages elimination, it's just as important for those without health issues as it is for people dealing with conditions that often come with aging—high cholesterol and blood sugar, certain cancers, bowel disorders, and even excess weight. For example, researchers at the University of California, Davis, found that adding fiber or fat to a low-fat, low-fiber diet increased levels of a hormone associated with feelings of hunger satisfaction in women. In addition, fiber has fewer calories than fat, making it a smart addition to any weight loss plan.[10]

All fiber is plant-based and passes through our bodies undigested. But different kinds of fiber offer different benefits. The two best-known categories are *soluble* and *insoluble,* terms that indicate the fiber's ability to retain water. Soluble fiber can absorb lots of water, while insoluble fiber is less water retentive. When combined with water or another liquid, soluble fiber becomes gelatinous. This quality slows digestion, and helps regulate blood sugar as well as reduce hunger. On the other hand, insoluble fiber does not change as it passes through the intestines, which makes it useful for maintaining bowel regularity, among other things. The fiber in food is generally a combination of soluble and insoluble.

FIBER FACTS

In addition to insoluble and soluble fiber, there are other types, each providing different health benefits. These include bran, which includes gums and mucilages, cellulose, hemicellulose, lignin, and pectin.

The most famous fiber, bran, can lower cholesterol, and it's now added to some cereal, snacks, and bread. But read labels on these products carefully; some of them contain only a little bran and too much sugar, salt, and fat. You can also buy oat and wheat bran and use them for cooking and baking.

Cellulose and hemicelluose are insoluble fibers that are

excellent for intestinal cleansing. Apples, pears, broccoli, carrots, green beans, and peas are good sources of both these fibers.

Another type of fiber, lignin, is one of the reasons flaxseeds are rising stars in the health world. Lignin lowers cholesterol, and it is also thought to reduce the risk of certain types of cancer.

Eating apples, carrots, cabbage, and bananas provides several types of fiber, including cholesterol-lowering pectin. Diabetics or people with blood sugar irregularities benefit from pectin, because it keeps food in the stomach longer, avoiding insulin overload.

The American Dietetic Association recommends 20 to 35 grams of fiber daily for healthy adults, but the typical American consumes only about half this amount. Eating more whole foods is an easy way to get adequate amounts of fiber. Here's a partial list of foods high in fiber:

- Beans, including baked, kidney, black, pinto, lima, soy, and navy beans, plus legumes like peas and lentils
- Whole grains, brown rice, bran, and all-bran cereals
- Prunes, Asian pears, artichokes, raspberries, blackberries, boysenberries, mixed frozen vegetables, and dried fruits
- Air-popped, unbuttered popcorn; nuts and seeds
- Glucomannan, flaxseeds, and psyllium

You can check the fiber content of other foods at this government Web site: www.nal.usda.gov/fnic/etext/000020.html. Click on the "Reports by Single Nutrients" link to search for high-fiber fare.

Putting Fiber in Your Diet

Adding more fiber to your diet means swapping processed grains, like white bread, for whole grains, like whole-wheat bread. Begin by looking for a breakfast cereal that provides 8 to 10 grams of fiber per serving. If your LDL ("bad") cholesterol levels are high, try an oat cereal. Researchers at Colorado State University found that oat cereal decreased production of LDL cholesterol better than wheat cereal, without affecting HDL ("good") cholesterol levels.[11] Cutting cholesterol benefits the heart and supports good hearing.

Next, aim for one-half cup brown rice (about 2 grams of fiber) and one cup of beans (most beans have close to 15 grams of fiber in a cup) with lunch or dinner. Or load up on fruits and vegetables throughout the day. While most fruits and veggies have far less fiber than beans, they contain plenty of other healthful substances. Dried fruit is also a good choice. Dried figs, for example, have almost five times more fiber than the fresh version. Whole-grain cereals and breads, air-popped, unbuttered popcorn, legumes, nuts, and seeds are other excellent sources of fiber.

Quick Tips

The USDA dietary guidelines advise eating three or more daily servings of whole grains. A serving is defined as one ounce of grains or one slice of whole-wheat bread, so make sandwiches with whole-wheat bread to increase fiber intake. Increase the amount of fiber in your diet gradually, however, or you may experience bloating and gas. And boost water intake, especially if you use fiber supplements, to maintain regularity. Looking for an easy way to get more fiber? Try nuts. Rich in fiber, good fats, and antioxidants, nuts of all types (in moderation!) are a healthful addition to the diet.

Walnuts contain not only essential fatty acids but the antioxidant melatonin as well, making them doubly good for you.

PEANUTS: GOOD FATS, VITAMINS, AND MORE

Researchers at Pennsylvania State University have found that a daily serving of peanuts is a simple way to add good fats to the diet. Technically a legume, peanuts are excellent sources of fiber, and also contain such key nutrients as vitamins A, C, and E, plus calcium, magnesium, selenium, and potassium. No wonder they are sometimes called Mother Nature's vitamin pill.

Furthermore, the researchers report that individuals who ate moderate amounts of peanuts regularly tended to be leaner and have lower levels of saturated fats and cholesterol in their meals than people who did not consume peanuts.[12] There have been similar positive findings from research on almonds, as well as walnuts.

One serving of peanuts equals a one-ounce portion, while two tablespoons of peanut butter constitute a serving.

Look for natural peanut butter, rather than the conventional variety. The natural version is made only of peanuts (with or without salt). It requires refrigeration, but it provides far more nutrients and good, monounsaturated and polyunsaturated fats.

Getting to Know the Good Fats

One area of nutrition where confusion reigns is fat. Twenty-some years ago, fat was declared the enemy. Since then, attitudes have changed. Today, scientists have thorough documentation showing that the *type* of fat is what determines whether or not it is healthful. The so-called good fats are from the family of substances known as essential fatty acids (EFAs), and these, we now know, are helpful for protecting against a variety of conditions, including heart disease, stroke, depression, and attention-deficit hyperactivity disorder (ADHD).

As you can tell from their name, the EFAs are absolutely essential for good health. Our bodies can't produce them, however, so these fats must be obtained from food or supplements. The EFAs fall into two categories: omega-3s and omega-6s. Both types of EFAs play a role in a long list of important processes within the body, including creating new cells and repairing old ones, mental and nervous system functions, and emotional and heart health. We need both omega-3s and omega-6s to stay in top health, but we don't need a great amount of either one. The key to getting the most benefit from these EFAs is a properly balanced intake of both.

Ideally, the ratio of omega-3s to omega-6s is 3:1, which would parallel the diet humans ate as they evolved. Early humans relied on food sources like berries, greens, nuts, seeds, and roots, along with plant-fed animals. The food they ate contained far more of the omega-3 fatty acids than we consume today. Modern-day food is loaded with omega-6 fatty acids found in safflower, sunflower, soy, corn, and partially hydrogenated fats. As a result, the Standard American Diet's current ratio of omega-6s to omega-3s is approximately 20:1, far out of line with what nature intended.

There are several different types of omega-3s, including alpha-linolenic acid (ALA, not to be confused with the antioxidant alpha-lipoic acid), docosahexaenoic acid (DHA), and eicosapentaenoic acid (EPA).

Flax is the most abundant source of alpha-linolenic acid,

while DHA and EPA are found in fatty fish, like cod, salmon, sardines, mackerel, tuna, halibut, sea bass, and anchovies. One of the most dramatic examples of the extensive health benefits provided by the omega-3s comes from the follow-up research into the Lyon Diet Heart Study.

The researchers' purpose was to measure the ability of the so-called Mediterranean diet to reduce the risk of a second heart attack. Later in this chapter, there are more details on the Mediterranean diet, but for now here's an overview. The Mediterranean diet is built around fruits, vegetables, grains, fish, and good oils, like olive oil. The researchers tracked the health of approximately six hundred people and found that there was as much as a 70 percent reduction in second heart attacks among those who ate the Mediterranean diet.[13]

Similarly, dozens of clinical trials have underscored the importance of DHA and EPA found in fish oil. These oils are especially important for good heart health, because they minimize hardening of the arteries and can reduce triglyceride levels in the blood, while making blood platelets less likely to clump together and form a clot. Fish oil has also been shown to be helpful in regulating dangerous heart arrhythmias.

A look at two recent clinical trials shows how important fish oil can be in protecting against heart attacks, the nation's leading killer, for both men and women. The first study, involving 22,000 men, concluded that those with the highest levels of omega-3 fatty acids in their blood were a stunning 90 percent less likely to die suddenly from a heart attack.[14] The second study, part of the ongoing Nurses' Health Study involving nearly 90,000 women, found that those who consumed the most omega-3 fatty acids, either by eating fish or from supplements, had a lower risk of both heart disease and death from heart attacks.[15]

Flax: A Fish Oil Alternative?

The flax plant (*Linum usitatissimum*), which provides the raw material for linen, has a long history of medicinal use. Now the high content of omega-3 EFAs in flaxseeds and flax oil is making it an increasingly popular choice for anyone who wants to avoid fish. Be aware, however, that the oil found in flax is not, strictly speaking, the same as fish oil.

First, there is some controversy as to whether or not the body can effectively convert flax's ALA to EPA and DHA. Although in theory this should not be a problem, the process is not clearly established, and aging may reduce the body's ability to make the conversion.

There is no doubt that flaxseeds and flax oil have distinct health benefits, and many of these are shared with fish oil. For example, research has shown that flax can reduce risk factors for heart disease, by lowering high blood pressure, decreasing LDL cholesterol and triglyceride levels, maintaining flexibility in arteries, and preventing the "stickiness" that causes blood platelets to form clots. So if you're a vegetarian or vegan, or simply can't stand to eat fish, flaxseeds or flax oil might be a worthwhile alternative. Just be aware that the jury is still out on this one, although it's likely that the good outweighs the bad.

Choosing the Right Fish

Levels of DHA and EPA vary, so not all fish provide the same benefits. Fatty fish—salmon, cod, herring, sardines, tuna, anchovies, and mackerel—are good sources, but the amount of omega-3s in a serving of fish depends on where the fish is from. Those in the wild eat plants rich in the omega-3s, so they are considered a better source of these oils than farm-raised fish that eat grains. Whichever you choose, you don't need much; a mere four ounces of fish, an amount that's about the size of a deck of playing cards, is considered one serving.

What about toxins in fish? This is probably the biggest downside of adding fish to the diet. Eating farmed salmon, for example, is certainly not risk-free, as a study from Indiana University's School of Public and Environmental Affairs demonstrated. After analyzing more than two metric tons of farmed and wild salmon from all over the world, the scientists found that farmed salmon had consistently higher levels of organochlorine contaminants than wild fish. Furthermore, the results also showed that farm-raised salmon from Europe were far more contaminated than those from North or South America. According to the study's risk analysis, eating heavily contaminated salmon could counteract the health benefits of the omega-3 essential fatty acids found in these fish.[16]

You can minimize these risks by asking either the supermarket manager or the waiter in a restaurant where the fish comes from. Public concern is even resulting in the source of fish being included on labels.

Toxins such as mercury and PCBs can be eliminated from fish oil supplements through a process known as molecular distillation, and this will be noted on the product label. Fish oil supplements generally contain 12 percent DHA and 18 percent EPA. The suggested dosage ranges from 3 to 10 grams daily, so follow the dosage instructions on the product you choose or consult your health care provider for appropriate dosage.

Unless a doctor advises it, be careful when consuming good-fat supplements if you are taking blood thinners, such as Coumadin (warfarin) or aspirin, have epilepsy or other seizure disorders, schizophrenia, diabetes, liver or kidney disease, hemophilia, or are pregnant or lactating. If you are having surgery soon, tell your physician about any EFA supplements you are taking; since these fats thin the blood, they should be stopped ten to fourteen days prior to surgery and can usually be taken again two to three days following surgery.

FISH IN A CAPSULE

Ben felt as though he was living on borrowed time, and with good reason. His father had died from a heart attack in his forties, and Ben was now approaching his fiftieth birthday. At the same time, he was overweight and his cholesterol levels were far above levels that are considered safe. To make matters worse, he was having a terrible time on the job because his hearing was deteriorating. Since he was a judge, Ben agreed with my suggestion to get a hearing aid. The next time I saw him, he acknowledged that he was coping with the courtroom situation much better now. But he admitted that his other problems were still a concern.

His cardiologist, he explained, had recommended statins, and Ben's cholesterol levels began diminishing. But he soon developed muscle aches and other side effects that signaled trouble. The doctor had no choice but to take him off the statins. I suggested Ben consult a nutritionist to improve his diet. Maybe his cholesterol could be managed with a few dietary changes and proper supplements.

Ben was discouraged. Although he agreed to try supplements, he really wasn't hopeful that they could improve the situation. Furthermore, he didn't want to be bothered with dietary changes. But he kept the appointment with the nutritionist, and in the end, he was glad. She noted that his existing diet was really not bad at all, and then recommended he eat more fish, a suggestion that made him wince. "Thanks but no thanks. I hate fish," he admitted. "Even the ones that don't taste like fish. There must be something else."

As a matter of fact, said the nutritionist, there was. Had he tried fish oil? Same benefits, no worries about having to eat something you don't like. So Ben tried fish oil supplements.

Later, Ben told me that at his next checkup with the cardiologist, his triglyceride and cholesterol levels were much improved. Furthermore, the arthritis in his knees wasn't bothering him so much, and he was walking two miles every evening, which enabled him to lose a few pounds. "But the strangest thing has happened," he said. "When I take my hearing aid off at night, I can sit in the den and hear our son practicing the piano at the other end of the house, which I haven't been able to do for a couple of years. I'm not ready to throw the hearing aid away just yet, but I'm surprised at how much difference a few small changes can make."

Quick Tips

Eating fish provides protection against colon cancer, according to the results of an American Cancer Society study that followed more than 148,000 men and women, while red meat and processed meats increase the likelihood of the disease.

Another way to improve the ratio of omega-3s and omega-6s in the diet is to minimize intake of foods containing omega-6 vegetable oils, like corn and safflower oils. Typically, these are found in chips, baked goods, prepared meals, and fast foods.

Also try using flaxseed oil in salad dressings or dips—but not for cooking, since heat converts the essential fatty acids into damaging free radicals. Flaxseeds, which provide good fats and fiber, can be mixed into yogurt, stews, soups, or cereal. The outer shell is difficult for humans to digest, though, so grind a small portion (a coffee bean grinder does the job) for immediate use and keep the rest refrigerated.

And make an effort to avoid trans-fatty acids (TFAs), also known as trans fats, usually identified on food ingredient labels as "partially hydrogenated" oils. The highly regarded Institute of Medicine, an independent scientific advisory board, has determined that there is no safe intake level of these chemically created substances. They have been linked to heart attacks and other health concerns. Snack foods, cookies, baked goods, and many other convenience products often contain trans-fatty acids.

Skip the Sweet Stuff

So much has been written about sugar that we can cut to the chase. The primary problem with sugar is that it contains little in the way of nutrition, and the foods with highest sugar content are generally not very healthful, either. It's hard to escape sugar, though, as Rob discovered when he decided to eliminate as much of it as possible from his diet.

After Rob nearly passed out while on the assembly line at work, he visited his doctor and discovered that he was prediabetic. Snacks, sodas, cookies, and convenience foods were a big part of Rob's daily diet. His father had developed diabetes later in life, so Rob decided to give up as much sugar as possible. At first, he missed the cookies and soda that he had snacked on at lunchtime and during his break. But after a week or so, he discovered that his son would often take a little container of applesauce mixed with cinnamon or berries to school in his lunch box, and Rob tried it. "I couldn't remember the last time I ate applesauce, but it just hit the spot—sweet, but not too sweet—and I didn't have to feel guilty about eating it. So I started taking all kinds of fruit to work."

At first, Rob's co-workers teased him about trading in his soft drinks for water and eating fruit instead of the usual candy bars. But during the next few months, they saw the potbelly Rob had been carrying around disappear, and the teasing stopped.

Of course, as Rob or anyone else who has seriously tried to give up sugar knows, it is not easy. Sugar is found in everything from pasta sauces to bread to salad dressings. To make matters worse, food manufacturers often list sugar by other names, such as "sucrose," "fructose," and "dextrose." Generally speaking, any ingredient with "-ose" at the end of its name is some type of sugar. Carefully reading ingredient labels is the best way to determine if it contains some form of sugar.

One place you are likely to find high sugar content is in low-fat desserts. Reducing the fat content generally affects a product's taste, so manufacturers increase the sugar to make the food more appealing to the taste buds. Next time those low-fat cookies start to look tempting, check the ingredient list. It's a safe bet that sugar is one of the first few ingredients, which means that while the cookies could be low in fat, they're high in calories because of the sugar content.

Sweet and Dangerous: How High-Fructose Corn Syrup Harms Your Health

For years, we have been warned about the dangers of eating too much saturated fat, and more recently, trans-fatty acids have become the dietary villain to avoid. Somehow, though, high-fructose corn syrup (HFCS) has managed to maintain a fairly low profile, which is a bit surprising.

HFCS sounds innocuous, but it is not. A synthetically created form of sugar, HFCS does not stimulate the secretion of insulin or two hormones that govern appetite management, ghrelin and leptin. This means that when you consume foods or beverages with HFCS in them, feelings of hunger are not eased. So the calories not only provide no nutrition, but they also provide no satisfaction, and you're likely to eat more.

Like sugar, HFCS is added to hundreds of foods, and it can be found in the unlikeliest of places—bread, fruit beverages, salad dressings, barbecue sauce, ketchup, and much more. Experts have determined that HFCS is now so frequently added to food that the average American consumes more than sixty pounds of it a year. There is an interesting parallel between HFCS and the current obesity epidemic, too. The steady increase of HFCS in food, which started in the 1960s, actually corresponds to the gradually expanding waistlines in this country.[17]

Excess weight is not the only problem associated with HFCS. Clinical trials have shown that diets rich in HFCS result in substantial increases in triglyceride levels, a risk factor for heart disease. Furthermore, many people cannot digest HFCS, a condition known as fructose intolerance. The symptoms, including bloating, gas, stomach cramps, "rumbly tummy," or diarrhea, can occur even with as small an amount as is found in a 12-ounce soda (about 39 grams).

This may be due to the fact that HFCS contains considerably more fructose than any actual food, including fruit. But even if you haven't experienced gastric problems after consuming HFCS, I encourage you to consume as little as possible. It offers no nutritional advantage, and the simple fact that it raises triglyceride levels could affect the heart and, for that reason, possibly hearing as well.

Finally, there's one more sugar-related area to look at, and that is artificial sweeteners. Here is the bottom line on these products: They are unlikely to help with weight loss. In fact, studies conducted several years ago found that artificial sugars wreak havoc with the body's fat storage system, stimulate carbohydrate cravings, and increase feelings of hunger.

A study conducted at the University of Texas, San Antonio, provides a perfect illustration. After observing more than one thousand men and women for eight years, researchers found that people who drank diet soda were more likely to be overweight than those who drank normal soda with sugar. Drinking one diet soda per day resulted in a 65 percent increase in the likelihood of being overweight, while drinking two or more diet or near-diet sodas (low-calorie versions with artificial sweeteners) increased the probability of being overweight even more! In other words, the more diet soda people were consuming, the greater the risk of being overweight.[18]

There are other health-related concerns about artificial sweeteners that we don't need to consider here. The bottom line is that less sugar—in all its many forms, and that includes substitutes—is part of the Save Your Hearing Now Program. Consuming large amounts of sugary foods is linked to obesity, diabetes, cardiovascular problems, and aging, all conditions that can contribute to hearing loss.

Quick Tips

Replace sodas and fruit-flavored beverages with water and add flavor (as well as antioxidants) with a wedge of citrus fruit or a slice of ginger.

Drink more tea—lots more. Studies consistently show that all types of tea—green, black, white, red, you name it—are loaded with antioxidants and other beneficial substances.

Can't live without something sweet? Satisfy craving with small amounts of chocolate. Pass on milk chocolate and choose the darkest varieties, which are rich in antioxidants known as polyphenols.

Making Moderation Work for You

Earlier, I mentioned that hundreds of studies have shown considerable health benefits from caloric restriction, which typically eliminates about one-third of the calories from the daily diet. For many people, this is a far too drastic measure. But making small reductions in the amount of food consumed is a simple, effective way to manage weight.

An eye-opening study from Penn State University shows how easy it is to let portion size get out of control. In this clinical trial, subjects were provided a macaroni and cheese lunch once each week for one month. The meals varied in size, ranging from 500 grams (more than one pound of pasta) to 1,000 grams, so even the smallest meal was actually quite hearty. But both men and women in the study ate a whopping 30 percent more of the 1,000-gram meal than they did when served the 500-gram meal. And most of them did not feel more satisfied with the larger amount of food. In fact, fewer than 50 percent of the participants even noticed the meals were different in size.[19] Similar studies on the effects of portion size at Cornell University and New York University have supported these findings.

What does this mean to someone who is trying to drop a few pounds? Those "super-sized" meals are your worst enemy. Use smaller plates to make portions look larger, eat slowly, put your fork down between bites, and chew food thoroughly—in other words, do whatever you have to do to cut back on the amount of food you are eating.

Furthermore, don't let dining out turn into an excuse for overeating. Restaurant portions these days are enormous— the equivalent of two or three meals in some cases, as restaurants try to survive in a highly competitive arena. So here's a suggestion: Split the entrée and even a salad, with a partner. Or if you're eating alone, ask the waiter to bring only half the meal and to wrap the other half to go before it even gets to the table. If it is not on your plate, you can't eat it all in one sitting.

How to Eat

By now, you should have a good idea of what kinds of foods to add to your diet to follow the Save Your Hearing Now Program. But *how* you eat is important, too, especially if you want to drop some pounds or improve overall health. Here are some suggestions:

Don't diet. Being on a diet suggests that at some point the diet will end. What usually happens then? The weight returns. This lose-weight, gain-weight pattern is known as yo-yo dieting, and it can affect metabolism negatively, as well as reduce levels of HDL ("good") cholesterol. Keeping levels of HDL cholesterol high is vitally important to good heart health, and therefore hearing as well.

Eat often. Divide the total number of calories for the day into more than three meals. Ideally, you should aim for five or six small meals throughout the day. The key word here: small. For the average person, this means no more than 250 to 300 calories at each mini-meal. This prevents you from becoming so hungry that you scarf down the first candy bar that crosses your path, and also supplies your body with a steady source of nutrients throughout the day.

Do not skip meals, especially breakfast. The human body is designed to survive in times when food is scarce, as it no doubt was for our prehistoric ancestors. So when you don't eat, the body goes into "starvation mode," and metabolism slows. If you're hoping to drop some pounds, a slow metabolism is not what you want. Additionally, a number of studies have found that eating breakfast helps reduce hunger pangs that can lead to overeating later in the day.

Do not buy into the "clean plate" mentality. If leaving food on your plate makes you feel guilty, start with one-half or one-third of what you would normally put on the plate.

Speaking of plates, downsize. Serve smaller portions on smaller plates so there's no sense of deprivation involved.

Stop eating before you feel full. It takes the brain about twenty minutes or so to recognize that the stomach is satisfied.

Eat fruit first. Start taking fresh fruit, ready-to-eat vegetables, or small packets of nuts with you to ward off hunger. If you eat a banana or half a grapefruit before lunch, the odds are you won't be so hungry when it's time to eat.

Read food labels. Devote some time to this, and you'll quickly see why most convenience foods are not recommended. For those who are in a time crunch, visit the local health food store and check out the freezer section. Generally, these products are much better than what you'll find in a supermarket's freezer, although some major chains are starting to offer more nutritious frozen fare.

Pop it! Buy an air popper and snack on air-popped popcorn, seasoned with a little butter-flavored spray and an herbal seasoning blend. Popcorn is high in fiber, and it satisfies the urge to nibble with fairly few calories.

De-stress with magnesium and more. If stress drives you to the refrigerator, magnesium-rich foods (nuts, whole grains, legumes, seeds, and veggies) can help tense muscles relax.

(Remember, magnesium also protects the ears from noise.) A small amount of unsalted sunflower seeds, an excellent source of the calming amino acid L-tryptophan, makes a good evening snack on stressful days.

Put veggies first. When you're planning meals, start with vegetables, then add whole grains, like brown rice, whole-wheat bread or pasta, with small amounts of low-fat dairy products and lean protein. Choose a good fat, like olive or grape-seed oil, for salads and dipping. Use fresh fruits to replace high-sugar desserts.

Now for the Don'ts

Do not buy junk food, candy, or sodas. If it is not in the house, you can't eat it.

Do not consume energy bars, meal replacement bars, and most sports drinks. Typically, these are loaded with sugar in one form or another. Remember, whole foods, whole foods, whole foods are your best source of nutrients.

Do not give up and revert to old habits if you feel you've made a "mistake." Who doesn't want to have the occasional slice of cheesecake at the office birthday party, or an extra helping of Mom's spaghetti? Life is short. If you enjoy something extra today, go for a longer walk tomorrow.

Do not weigh yourself more than once a week. Instead, let the fit of your clothes be your guide.

Do not use herbal weight loss products that contain stimulants. They can rev up the central nervous system and make people feel anxious and jumpy.

WEIGHT AND GENES

"I know I'm heavy, but my whole family is like this. There's nothing I can do about it." I hope this doesn't sound familiar, because you are doing yourself a disservice to claim that because your parents or other family members are overweight, you are doomed to carry extra pounds. Genes do play important roles in our health. But scientists are discovering that environment—in terms of how we live, eat, and exercise—is even more important.

Researchers in England, for example, studied more than four hundred children from families that were obese, overweight, normal weight, or lean. In taste tests, they found that children from the families with excess weight preferred fatty foods and were less interested in vegetables than the kids from average weight or lean families. In addition, overeating was more common in the obese/overweight group, as was a preference for sedentary activities. The researchers concluded that lifestyle choices passed on from parents to children, including preferred foods and a tendency toward low activity, could be part of the process of transmitting obesity to the next generation.[20]

How to Get There from Here

You're convinced you need to change your diet, but where do you begin? Clearly, you should plan to spend more time in the produce aisle. A good place to start: the USDA's recently released "food guidance system." Basically an overhaul of the old food pyramid, the new version is based on input from dozens of experts, many studies, public opinion, and, of course, food industry lobbyists. Most of the changes are geared toward helping people manage or lose weight. (The guidelines are available online at http://www.healthierus.gov/dietaryguidelines.)

Among other things, the new recommendations advise reducing sugar and salt intake, limiting saturated fats, choosing low-fat dairy products, and minimizing intake of trans fats, the partially hydrogenated vegetable oils found in many fast foods and processed snacks that are even worse for the body than saturated fats.

Furthermore, the experts now suggest *nine* or more servings of fruits and vegetables daily. (Sorry, but french fries and ketchup don't count.) Nine servings may sound like an impossible number. For many people, the old recommendation of five daily servings was overwhelming. But before you throw up your hands in despair, let's look at what that really means. A serving is technically defined as one-half cup. If you look at the half-cup line on your measuring cup, you'll see that a half cup isn't much— a handful of baby carrots, a few broccoli or cauliflower florets, several melon balls, and you're on your way.

Another great way to boost vegetable intake is based on research from Penn State University's Laboratory for the Study of Human Ingestive Behavior. Studies there have demonstrated that it is possible to eliminate 30 percent of a meal's calories by simply replacing high-calorie ingredients in pasta salads and casseroles with vegetables and still have a satisfying meal.

Subjects in one study ate both high-calorie and vegetable-rich meals on different days. Each time, they consumed roughly the same amount of food and reported the same satisfaction with both meals, so clearly, there were no feelings of deprivation involved with the higher-vegetable-intake meal.[21]

How do you put this information to use? One easy way is to make a dish like pasta primavera, a combination of pasta and vegetables, but use twice as many vegetables and half as much pasta as the recipe calls for. And be creative! If a recipe lists a vegetable you are not particularly fond of—let's say lima beans, for example—substitute another green veggie that you like, such as green beans, broccoli, or peas.

Here is another way to increase vegetable intake and reduce calorie intake at the same time. In a related study, the Penn State research team found that women who ate a low-calorie salad prior to a pasta lunch ate less pasta than the control group that was not served a salad. Not surprisingly, the larger the salad, the less pasta was eaten.[22] It's important to note, though, that the low-calorie salads were primarily greens and vegetables with low-fat dressing and very little cheese. In other words, salads drowning in dressing, croutons, cheese, and other high-calorie extras are not going to obtain the same results.

One way to raise veggie intake substantially is to turn your salad into a salad bar whenever possible. Supermarket shelves are now loaded with convenience packs of clean, ready-to-eat produce—shredded carrots and cabbage, sliced peppers, chopped, washed broccoli, and so on. Add some cherry or tiny pear tomatoes, artichoke hearts, olives, and a small amount of a simple dressing combining olive oil and lemon juice, and you have a meal that is satisfying and good for you.

If you get sick of salads, stores also offer prepared mixed greens that can be steamed with a small amount of water in just a minute or two. Drizzle on a little olive oil, season with your favorite spices—roasted, minced garlic is a nice, healthful addition—and you're done!

Researchers point to the fact that vegetables, fruits, low-fat dairy products, cooked whole grains, stews, and soups are less "energy dense" (i.e., contain fewer calories) than pasta or meat because they contain a higher proportion of water. This higher water intake contributes to post-meal satisfaction. So by starting with a big, fresh salad or increasing the amount of vegetables in a dish like pasta primavera, for example, it's possible to significantly reduce calories without sacrificing flavor or satisfaction.

Homemade vegetable and/or bean soups, not the canned variety, are other great options. Make a big pot on the weekend and freeze small portions for later in the week. I like the version of vegetable soup that incorporates pesto. The basil and olive oil are not only healthful choices, they add a tremendous amount of flavor to the soup. Just remember to use sparingly. Start with a teaspoon stirred into a bowl of hearty soup and add a little more if necessary. To avoid overdoing it with olive oil, add a quarter cup or so of freshly chopped basil leaves and only a bit of pesto.

The Mediterranean Diet: Where Taste and Nutrition Meet

The Mediterranean diet has been studied all over the world by nutrition experts at major universities and found to deliver outstanding benefits for heart health. As we have mentioned before, good hearing requires good circulation, so eating for a healthy heart also helps the auditory system.

The Mediterranean diet is based on vegetables, fruits, whole grains, nuts, lean protein (generally, eggs, fish, or chicken), a little cheese or other low-fat dairy foods, and good fats, like olive oil. Many experts add a daily glass or two of wine as well, although that's an individual matter. High-quality, organic grape juice is a good, nonalcoholic option.

The Mediterranean diet has an important advantage over many other eating plans because it's exceptionally tasty, flexible, and not nearly as restrictive as some other approaches, so it works well for people who don't like to be hungry. Furthermore, there's a good chance of increasing longevity by switching to this eating plan. According to a recent decade-long study in the *Journal of the American Medical Association* (*JAMA*), adults between the ages of seventy and ninety who followed the Mediterranean diet slashed their risk of dying from heart disease, cancer, and other causes by 23 percent.[23]

Rebecca, a patient who tried the Mediterranean diet along with the program's other lifestyle changes, reported an interesting benefit that occurred after she changed her eating habits. As she explains it, working as a nurse in a pediatrician's office means being exposed to an endless number of bacteria and viruses every day. "I used to be sick pretty much all year, but winters were the worst—just one cold or flu after another," she says. "And every time I got congested, my hearing became even worse because my ears were so stuffy. I tried one cold medicine after another, but they either made me sleepy or dehydrated, or they just didn't work."

When she switched to fresh fruits and vegetables, though, Rebecca began eating much more raw produce than ever before. "It was so easy to pick up a ready-made salad of chopped raw vegetables or prepared fruit at the market," she explains. "So every day, I had my fresh, raw food for lunch."

Rebecca didn't even notice that she had been cold-free for several months until she went on a skiing trip, leaving behind her supplements and resuming her old eating habits. Within a couple of days, she came down with a cold and had to spend the week with stuffy ears. "When I came home and went back to work, I started the supplements again and got back into the salad routine. A couple of weeks later, I realized that even though there were some nasty bugs out there and everyone else was sick, I was fine. No cold, no stuffy ears. So I tell everyone, forget the cold medicine—take your vitamins, eat smart, and you won't need it."

EGGS AID IN WEIGHT LOSS

According to a new report in the *Journal of the American College of Nutrition,* the high-quality protein found in eggs may help win the battle of the bulge. Researchers tested two different 1,700-calorie diets in a group of middle-aged women. The high-protein version included a breakfast built around eggs, lean meat, and low-fat dairy products, while the other contained higher levels of carbohydrates.

After ten weeks, both groups had lost similar amounts of weight. But in the protein group, nearly twice as much of the weight loss was fat, while the carbohydrate group lost fat and muscle. One key difference between the diets was the amount of leucine, a branched-chain amino acid, that each contained. The high-protein diet contained twice as much leucine, found in eggs, and researchers note that the amino acid has been shown to affect metabolism in ways that can enhance fat loss.[24] Incidentally, eggs are an important element in the Mediterranean diet, according to a study from Spain.[25]

In the very near future, a new field known as nutritional genomics, or nutra-genomics, will make it possible for custom-designed meal plans to enhance our natural, genetic strengths and minimize our inherent weaknesses. Somehow, though, I don't think we are likely to see hot fudge sundaes replacing fruits and vegetables on anyone's healthful foods list. The sooner you begin making better food choices, the greater the chance that your hearing and health will benefit.

The Save Your Hearing Now Program is a good place to begin revamping your diet, because the recommendations are all designed to provide nutrition that supports better hearing. If weight is an issue, the combination of "less food, more activity" is one of the most effective weight loss strategies available, and I highly recommend this commonsense approach to anyone with a weight management problem. It's not trendy or glamorous, but it works. But we need to clarify one thing: When I say "less food," what I really mean is less bad food. If you're exercising, you can actually eat more, as long as you focus on the right foods. It is important to recognize, though, that exercise is for everyone, no matter what you weigh. In the following chapter, we will look at why exercise is so important and how it protects hearing.

((8))

STEP THREE: MOVE IT!

Deidre and Allen had a long history of involvement in music, he as a cellist with a regional symphony and she as a professional pianist and university music professor. Not surprisingly, both developed hearing difficulties in their mid-fifties. Deidre had to repeatedly ask students to speak up, and Allen found that he was losing interest in social events because he had to pretend to be able to hear conversations. "I always enjoyed a good give-and-take with friends about current events, politics, movies, sports, and what have you," he explained. "But now I can't hear well enough to take part."

Both Deidre and Allen enthusiastically decided to try the Save Your Hearing Now Program, but while Allen enjoyed the exercise aspect, Deidre did not. "It's just not me," she complained. "I'm not a jumping-around kind of person."

Allen's hearing deterioration eased after a few months, to the point where he was once again able to take part in conversations in social settings. But Deidre did not experience the same benefits. Frustrated, she considered giving up. But during a consultation, I mentioned that the exercise component might be all she needed to achieve success. The enhanced circulation from moderate physical activity could be what was needed to better distribute the nutrients from food and supplements. Why not try it?

Deidre agreed only because she had already benefited from the program in terms of weight loss, and she was enjoying the food. Moreover, Allen's success encouraged her. So she mapped out a short walk through the nearby mall, which would enable her to avoid being exposed to the coming winter weather. "At first," she recalls, "nothing happened. But once I got in the habit, I enjoyed walking every day. Several neighbors joined me, and it became a nice, early morning get-together."

Winter turned into spring and then summer before Deidre noticed that her hearing was different. "Actually, I didn't notice it, but one of my students did," she recalls. "He told me it was nice that he didn't have to keep repeating questions, and I thought, 'Why, he's right. I think I'll keep taking those walks.'"

Do Something Different

Visit the average gym, and you'll see people who are either thoroughly bored or so grimly determined to put in their mandatory time on the treadmill that they have to grit their teeth to do it. Who wants to spend even a few minutes of free time like that?

Human beings are made to move, but I hesitate to recommend that anyone do something each and every day they don't like doing. So find something you enjoy. Actually, find a few different pleasant activities so you can avoid the inevitable injuries that come with repetitive motions. Like a varied diet, varied exercise is more appealing, and it prevents boredom and injury too.

Here is another reason to put variety into exercise: Good

fitness has three different aspects—cardiovascular conditioning, stretching, and muscle building. Ideally, a workout program incorporates all three of these. While aerobic exercise, like brisk walking, is excellent for strengthening the cardiovascular system and for burning calories, weight training is important for maintaining muscles that are essential for good balance and bone health. Stretching helps prepare muscles for exercise and allows them to relax afterward, so there is less chance of injury or soreness.

Quick Tips

If you like to exercise with music, keep the volume low. And take earplugs to aerobics classes. The dB levels of the music played during aerobics classes can register well above the high 90s.[1]

Water is the preferred thirst quencher, for before, during, and after a workout. If you exercise intensely and/or sweat heavily, sports drinks can replace lost electrolytes. But choose a beverage that does not contain high-fructose corn syrup.

Why Everyone Should Get Moving

From the perspective of improved hearing, physical activity provides the obvious benefits of better heart health, weight management, and a reduction in the damage associated with aging. Furthermore, since circulation is increased, flow of oxygen and nutrients into the ear and brain are enhanced. But there is another important consideration. People who are in good shape are more likely to be healthy overall, and that fact alone reduces the risk of being prescribed an ototoxic drug.

Here is another consideration: Physical activity can help you save money. CDC experts worked out on their number crunchers and calculated that regular exercise could save Americans a grand total of more than $76 billion each year in health care costs. And there is further proof that activity pays off: Fit individuals save about $330 in medical expenses annually when compared with the sedentary.

How Working Out Helps Your Heart and Your Hearing

The most significant link between exercise and improved hearing is strengthening the heart. Any muscle becomes stronger when it is exercised, and the heart, which is a muscle, is no exception. With a strong, healthy heart, circulation improves, allowing oxygen and important nutrients to be delivered more effectively throughout the body and brain, where a good portion of the auditory system is located.

Aerobic exercise—any activity that makes the heart beat faster—provides the greatest benefits to the cardiovascular system. Walking, hiking, running, swimming, cycling, dancing, jumping rope, rock climbing, kayaking, and some forms of yoga qualify as aerobic exercise. Regular sessions of aerobic activity are the best way to keep your heart strong. Ideally, that means spending at least a half hour (more is better!) working out five or six days a week. Keep in mind, though, that a little exercise is better than none. If you only have ten minutes to spare, go for it.

Exercise experts recommend that sedentary individuals start with a short workout—twenty minutes, for example, every other day—and work up to longer sessions. Of course, if you have been sedentary, have any chronic health condition, or are under a physician's care, discuss starting an exercise program with your doctor beforehand.

Quick Tips

If you are not able to carry on a conversation during an aerobic workout because you are too out of breath, slow down—you're working too hard.

Exercise of any kind improves health, but aerobic exercise is the best when it comes to strengthening the heart. Experts agree that one way to improve heart health is to raise levels of HDL ("good") cholesterol. Exercise can help accomplish this, but only if you burn off roughly 1,200 calories per week. Using walking as an example, taking a brisk hike at least four times each week and covering three miles should do it.

Explore the Exercise Options

Walking is a good foundation for a workout program. Aim for some walking time—say, thirty minutes a day—then build on that with stretching (yoga or Pilates, for example) and strength training. There is an ever-growing number of possibilities when it comes to working out, as fitness professionals strive to keep people interested and motivated. If money is no object, visit a shop that specializes in home gym equipment, and you'll very likely be surprised at the sophistication of today's treadmills, elliptical trainers, step machines, and stationary cycles. Some models come with video screens that can be programmed to display different landscapes, so you can imagine you're cycling through the south of France or another favorite destination, while others are Internet-ready and capable of relaying performance feedback from the manufacturer's Web site. Most also have some method of measuring heart rate, and more, during activity.

Of course, many people don't have thousands of dollars to plunk down on a stair climber, but that's one nice thing about this market. Many people buy exercise equipment and find that they aren't using it, so it's possible to pick up a used (but not much!) model for a lot less than the original price. Check the local classified ads or the yellow pages, since there are stores that specialize in reselling exercise equipment.

If you prefer the companionship of other exercisers, gyms or the YWCA or YMCA are generally well equipped and loaded with classes in everything from aerobics to yoga.

The Exercise Connection to Weight Management

Earlier, we discussed the obesity epidemic and noted that more than 60 percent of the adults in the United States are considered overweight or obese. As a result, these individuals' overall health and hearing are compromised. Fortunately, exercise can help with weight management. Losing weight is not simply a matter of eating less. In fact, most health experts believe dieting is only part of the story when it comes to managing weight. Without physical activity of some sort, diets often do more harm than good.

The bottom line with any diet is deprivation. You're giving up something—bread, dessert, candy, alcohol, second helpings, whatever—and that's no fun. The great thing about exercise is that it raises endorphin levels, those feel-good hormones that provide a "runner's high." Endorphins can help eliminate any feelings of self-pity caused by passing on that double-fudge brownie or second helping of mashed potatoes. Exercise also boosts the metabolism, thereby increasing energy and making it easier to lose weight. How many calories were in that brownie—about 130? An extra thirty-five minutes of brisk walking burns about that many calories, so it may be possible to have your brownie and eat it, too, if you're willing to spend more time being active. And there's the added benefit of just feeling good about doing something you know is healthy.

As we noted in Chapter Seven, the Departments of Agriculture and Health and Human Services recently updated the national dietary guidelines, with an emphasis on cutting back on calories and increasing regular exercise. The biggest change is in the exercise guidelines. If your weight is appropriate, the old thirty-minutes-per-day recommendation is adequate, although sixty minutes most days of the week is even better when it comes to strengthening the heart and maintaining muscle.

But if you want to shed some pounds, the federal government experts suggest going further and getting sixty to ninety minutes of activity daily. In addition, they emphasize that children and teens stay active for sixty minutes a day, double the amount of time formerly recommended.

Sixty to ninety minutes a day may sound like an awful lot of exercise, especially for anyone who is sedentary and spending zero minutes working out now. But keep one thing in mind: The minutes do not have to occur all at the same time. Several studies have shown that dividing total exercise time into two, three, or four segments each day effectively delivers the same health benefits as one longer session. An added bonus: Divvying up exercise throughout the day may result in more calories being burned than one prolonged session.

Exercise does not necessarily mean spending hours at the gym with a personal trainer. If a treadmill, stationary bicycle, or elliptical trainer would strap your budget, try a small trampoline. Park it in front of the television and use it while you watch your favorite shows. If that's out of reach, too, you can always walk in place in front of the TV. Add an exercise mat or folded-up blanket on the floor for some stretching and abdominal crunches, and you're on your way. The thing that's especially useful about this approach is that bad weather does not give you an excuse to stop working out. In other words, there's no excuse for being sedentary when exercise has so many proven health benefits. If you prefer going outside, you gain the advantages of variety and a change of scenery. Remember, moderate exercise—walking, gardening, dancing, swimming, tai chi—is fine, just so long as you get moving!

PEDOMETERS STEP UP FITNESS

In the mid-1960s, when the Olympic Games were held in Tokyo, a physical fitness craze swept Japan. At about the same time, pedometers, simple motion-sensor devices that count an individual's footsteps, went on the market. The result was a national passion for walking with a pedometer, with a daily goal of 10,000 steps for good health. The craze turned into a lifestyle. Now more than 7 million pedometers are sold in Japan every year, and *manpo-kei*—Japanese for "10,000 steps meter"—is the slogan adopted by thousands of walking clubs.

Now pedometers are gaining a foothold in the United States. The results of recent studies show that these simple, inexpensive devices can be helpful for anyone aiming to become more active. Based on current evidence relating to fitness and health, one group of experts at Arizona State University identified five levels to use as targets for pedometer-based fitness:

1. Less than 5,000 steps per day is considered "sedentary."
2. 5,000 to 7,499 steps per day is classified as "low active."
3. 7,500 to 9,999 is defined as "somewhat active."
4. "Active" individuals are those who take more than 10,000 steps daily.

5. Anyone walking more than 12,500 steps daily falls into the "highly active" category.

Using these guidelines and a simple pedometer, it is easy to measure your current level of activity and "take steps," so to speak, to increase it accordingly.[2]

Does the simple act of wearing a pedometer really increase activity levels, though? The results of several studies show that the answer to that question is yes. In one, a team of health experts from the University of Minnesota found that pedometers were a good way to keep people moving. They briefed a group of nearly one hundred inactive individuals on the importance of exercise, with a short lecture and printed handout. About half were also given pedometers and asked to keep activity logs. After two months, researchers examined both groups. Physical activity had increased in both, but the individuals in the pedometer group were most active, adding roughly twenty minutes of walking to each day.[3] Those findings were supported by a similar study involving only women at the University of Tennessee. Pedometers start at about twenty dollars, making these devices small investments with big payoffs.

Quick Tips

Find out how many calories your favorite activities burn at this Web site: http://www.calorieking.com, where you'll also find plenty of information on food, weight management, and nutrition.

Tai chi, a gentle, low-impact form of exercise developed centuries ago in China, can help older individuals improve their sense of balance, thereby preventing dangerous falls. A recent study reported that older people who practiced tai chi had a 50 percent reduction in risk of falling compared to those who did not.[4]

Put a spare pair of comfortable shoes in your car or at work, for those times when you have an extra fifteen or twenty minutes of downtime. Then there's no excuse for not using the time to take a walk.

Exercise Is for Everyone

Before we go further, there are two more points to make in regard to exercise. First, regardless of your weight, physical activity is extremely important. Simply being thin or having a BMI in the normal range does not, in and of itself, indicate good health. Because exercise strengthens the cardiovascular system and stimulates circulation, being sedentary puts hearing at risk in the same way as being obese. So even if you're slender, get moving!

Second, if you're exercising to encourage weight loss, don't skip meals. As we mentioned earlier, our national obsession with dieting is actually a major contributing factor to weight gain. Here's why: When the body is deprived of nutrition—say, a skipped breakfast, or even a hearty lunch of processed, nutritionless junk food—it obtains energy from its emergency reserves, which are stored in lean muscle tissue.

As the amount of muscle tissue in the body decreases, so do the number of calories burned at rest. So the body is burning off less food, and the muscles are weakened, making muscle-building, strenuous exercise difficult. Weight gain occurs. Dieting continues. The body is getting even less nutrition, and so it consumes more muscle tissue. This vicious cycle of muscle loss and weight gain can continue indefinitely, with disastrous results. As muscles weaken, body fat continues to accumulate, until it eventually interferes with an individual's ability to perform everyday tasks. And there's another complication: Muscle tissue burns many more calories than fat, even at rest. So by sitting around and letting muscles weaken, you're losing one of the best fat-burners ever invented!

Age Better by Building Muscle

While we are on the subject of muscles, let's spend a few minutes looking at one element of exercise that needs to be emphasized: Strength training. Frequently, people avoid this aspect of working out, because they are worried that weights will turn them into the Incredible Hulk. Trust me, with the type of weight training we are talking about, that won't happen. Bodybuilders go to extreme lengths to achieve those results, involving measures that are too drastic for the average person to endure. Fortunately, focusing on strength training for twenty or forty minutes two or three times a week will not create a bodybuilder's physique.

It will, however, tone the muscles, help maintain strong bones, and provide the strength and stability to grow old gracefully and in good health. You don't need a gym membership or fancy equipment to take advantage of the benefits of strength training; small free weights or even inexpensive "resistance bands" that look like giant rubber bands are fine, and, again, you can work out while watching television or talking on the phone.

Stronger muscles play a major role in healthy aging. As the years pass, our bodies undergo a series of changes. One of those is the loss of bone, a condition known as *osteoporosis*. While osteoporosis has received a great deal of publicity, few people are aware of another condition that is just as serious—*sarcopenia* (sar-ko-peen-ya). Sarcopenia was named by the CDC as one of the five greatest threats to healthy aging, but in spite of that, it is far from a household word.

While osteoporosis weakens the bones, sarcopenia weakens the muscles. Lean muscle starts to diminish sometime during early adulthood. By the time an individual reaches the middle years, muscle deterioration is ongoing; on average, adults over the age of forty are losing muscle at the rate of one-quarter to one-third of a pound annually. At the same time, there is an increase in body fat of roughly the same amount. Essentially, sarcopenia is the process of trading muscle for fat, and it is a prime factor behind the high levels of body fat in older people. (Remember, muscle is an outstanding calorie-burner, so this loss of muscle during middle age no doubt contributes to the bulge many people battle during this time of life.)

The danger of sarcopenia is not so much from the weight itself, although extra pounds are clearly not good for you. The problem is that the muscles become too weak to support the body, thus increasing the likelihood of falls and broken bones in older individuals.

How does sarcopenia affect hearing? People who feel weak are more likely to be sedentary, so circulation is poor. In addition, the added weight that can accumulate further robs people of movement, and as we saw earlier, excess pounds can accelerate aging and damage the brain. Healthy aging means staying active, and that requires muscles that are capable of supporting everyday functions. Hearing benefits from movement, as does the entire body. So please don't ignore strength training. It may not strengthen your hearing directly, but it plays a major supportive role.

Quick Tips

Building muscle can help manage blood pressure. Research at Medical College of Georgia found that blood pressure readings among people with more lean muscle tissue than fat returned to normal more quickly after a stressful event than did those in a group of people with higher body fat levels.

When lifting weights, start small (two or five pounds) and

add more repetitions (between eight and fifteen) rather than weight to strengthen muscles without "bulking up."

When performing strength-training exercises, don't race. Slow, steady moves accomplish more than rapid repetitions.

Exercise has benefits for every age group. If you have not been active and would like to begin, remember to start with a visit to your physician. Then explore some of the many exercise possibilities that are available. Gyms generally offer a wide selection of classes and instructors, but if you're not ready to go work out in public, there are plenty of books on exercise, so the local bookstore or library is an excellent place to start. In addition, video stores generally have shelves filled with videos and DVDs by popular exercise instructors that run the gamut from aerobics to yoga. Or you can work out with one of the dozens of television programs focusing on exercise instruction.

Finally, keep in mind you're never too old to gain benefits from physical activity. A good place to begin is by ordering a free copy of "Exercise: A Guide from the National Institute on Aging" by calling the toll-free number 800-222-2225. Animated exercises suitable for older people are available online at the NIA Web site: http://www.nih.gov/nia.

((**9**))

STEP FOUR: ALL ABOUT EAR PROTECTION

The Save Your Hearing Now Program is the foundation of good hearing. It begins with the supplements and lifestyle changes we have already discussed, but it does not end there. Minimizing the amount of noise in your life and protecting your ears from noise that cannot be escaped are the fourth element of the program. There are a variety of choices when it comes to ear protection, including earplugs and earmuffs. We will also look at noise-canceling headphones and white-noise devices, which do not technically protect the ears, but are useful for counteracting loud or annoying sounds.

Many patients ask when ear protection is appropriate. My answer is that ear protection should be used whenever you are exposed to loud noise of any kind. Remember, there is very little difference between the roar of a lawn mower, the whine of a power saw, the bone-thumping bass of the latest popular music, or a blow-dryer set on high in terms of how these sounds affect your ears. If you have experienced some hearing loss or are concerned about your continued high levels of noise exposure, invest in earplugs. They are tiny enough to be carried everywhere, as opposed to earmuffs, and they are easy to use.

The Ins and Outs of Earplugs

Inexpensive and easy to use, earplugs can protect against some noises, although they are not as effective as earmuffs. Today, earplugs are available in disposable foam models and one-size-fits-all molded plastic versions that are reusable, although they should be cleaned between wearings to eliminate bacteria that can cause ear infections. The molded plugs may seem more solid, but they do not fit in the ear as well as the disposable foam variety. For a little more money, however, you can get custom-fitted earplugs, based on molds made from your own ears, which avoid this problem.

Until recently, earplugs' big shortcoming was that once they were in place, they tended to muffle high-frequency sounds, so a musician, for example, wouldn't be able to hear very accurately. Today, though, there are high-tech earplugs that reduce loudness without distorting the sound. Instead of eliminating high frequencies, which is how standard earplugs work, these new earplugs "lower the volume." The wearer can hear high, low, and in-between sounds, without jeopardizing hearing, so they're useful for live-music performances or rehearsals, for example, as well as movies, sporting events, and other noisy activities.

One caution about earplugs: They may contribute to problems with earwax, because the plugs have to be "stuffed" into the ear. (By the way, do not—I repeat, do *not*—try to use cotton balls to protect your ears. Cotton is completely ineffective at protecting against noise. It reduces sound by a mere 5 to 7 dB and has the added downside of forcing earwax back against the eardrum.)

Earplugs are tested for effectiveness, and the resulting rating is shown on the package as Noise Reduction Rating (NRR). Plugs with a high NRR number provide more protection than a pair with a lower NRR. The NRR is expressed in decibels, so plugs with an NRR of 30 block out a maximum of 30 dB of sound. This maximum level, however, depends on a perfect fit and proper insertion. More typically, expect to obtain about half the amount of protection stated in the NRR. In other words, plugs with an NRR of 30 eliminate about 15 dB of noise. People who spend time in very noisy environments sometimes combine earplugs with earmuffs for maximum protection.

Basic earplugs are very inexpensive, often costing just pennies apiece, and they are available in many drugstores, at sporting goods stores, and from online retailers. Another nice feature of earplugs is that they fit in a pocket or purse, so there is no excuse for not taking them with you. People with longer hair can wear these without anyone noticing, too, which is sometimes a plus. Custom earplugs are also available; check with your audiologist or ENT for recommendations.

Often, patients say they are embarrassed to use earplugs. "The other guys will think I'm a big baby," confided a construction worker who was losing his hearing because of workplace noise. Of course, men aren't the only ones who are concerned about what people will think. Earplugs are close to hearing aids in appearance, and there is considerable stigma attached to both. In our culture, no one says, "Oh, she wears glasses. What a geezer!" Yet somehow hearing problems are considered far more embarrassing than changes in vision. Frankly, this attitude is just plain silly. I encourage patients to be completely open about the fact that they are protecting their hearing. Of course, it's not always easy, but keep in mind that hearing loss is no more a sign of weakness or frailty than being nearsighted. If, however, you're not comfortable discussing hearing loss, simply say that you are wearing ear protection because loud noises hurt your ears, and leave it at that.

WORKING AROUND NOISE

As we have seen, noise is virtually unavoidable in today's world. One method of coping is to block the noise with various devices. Another is to work during odd hours, when the world tends to be quieter. Mike, a self-employed accountant in San Diego, California, worked from his home quite happily for a number of years. That came to an end when a family with four young children moved in next door. As soon as the kids came home from school, they were in the yard, pounding a basketball on the pavement or clattering over the skateboard ramp their father had built. Mike's home office was only a few feet from this family's property line. When the noise became too distracting for him to concentrate, he spoke to the parents about the situation, but they were not interested in helping with his problem.

Mike's solution? He began getting up earlier, so he was able to complete eight or so hours of work by the time the kids came home in the late afternoon. During the hours they were playing in the backyard, he ran errands, visited friends, or finished up some less demanding chores in another part of the house.

Although Mike's situation involved neighborhood noise, people in business settings sometimes come in early or stay late as a way of escaping the noisiest and most distracting hours of the day. Sitting at your desk for an hour or two without phone or visitor interruptions can be very productive, in part because noise levels are much lower during early and late hours. Another way of implementing this approach involves blocking a period of "quiet time" into the day. This tactic is difficult to pull off without an office door to shut, but even if you work in a cubicle, you may be able to put the phone on voice mail and hang up a sign asking visitors to come back later.

Cover the Bases with Earmuffs

Unlike earplugs, earmuffs are hard to conceal. Not so long ago, the only models available couldn't be worn with any kind of hat, including hard hats, or with glasses. Another downside was that they tended to block out all types of sound, so it was impossible to hear speech, a real problem in work settings where people have to talk to one another.

Today, earmuffs are vastly improved, making them one of the best solutions for protecting ears from noise. New models are available that incorporate hard hats, while others feature noise reduction with communication (speech) amplifications, so conversation is possible while wearing the earmuffs. (Typical voice frequencies are amplified, but other loud sounds are dampened.) There are even earmuffs that block loud noise but allow the wearer to hear AM or FM radio. Adjustable, padded headbands and very lightweight models (less than six ounces) are also on the market. There are probably even more sophisticated features now offered in earmuffs, but as you can see, there really is something for everyone.

If you shop around, you can find earmuffs for less than ten dollars, and some retailers give discounts for multiple purchases. Earmuffs can be purchased at sporting goods stores or from retailers selling construction, farm, or safety accessories. Plenty of online retailers are selling hearing protection too. Just go to your favorite search engine and type in "hearing protection," "earmuffs," or "earplugs" to see what's available. If you've never worn this type of thing before, I suggest making a trip to a local store and trying on several pairs. This way you can find a good fit and a model you like, which obviously can't be done online.

Listen to the Music—or Not— with Noise-Canceling Headphones

Here's a common scenario: There's an annoying noise in the background, from a gardener's leaf blower, for example. It's not particularly loud, but that's not the issue. It's there. It is distracting. Actually, it's maddening. What to do?

Many people have found relief from this type of annoyance with noise-canceling headphones. Unlike earplugs or earmuffs, these devices do not protect the ears per se. Their purpose is to minimize background noise so that personal music players, like the iPod, can be heard in noisy settings, such as on airplanes or in subways. They come with a cord that can be plugged into the music player.

Noise-canceling headphones have another purpose, however. Since they emit a low-level white noise, these headphones mask bothersome background sounds. When a neighbor began construction my co-author, Marie Moneysmith, discovered how useful noise-canceling headphones can be while working on this book. The noise was not particularly loud in her office, but between the whining saws, banging hammers, and workers shouting at one another, concentration was difficult at best. Fortunately, she discovered that noise-canceling headphones dampened the construction sounds but allowed normal conversation—and concentration!

Other people have mentioned using noise-canceling headphones to get to sleep on an airplane, to save their sanity when a child was learning to play a musical instrument, and to study in libraries, which are no longer the oases of silence they once were.

Noise-canceling headphones are not rated for noise reduction (NRR). There are quite a few different models available, with prices ranging from a few dollars to hundreds. The most expensive ones are designed for audiophiles who demand excellent music quality. If you are only interested in the white-noise aspect, there's no need to spend a great deal. Noise-canceling headphones are available from some electronics and music retailers, as well as online.

The Sounds of Silence: An Easy Way to Protect Your Ears

Here's an often overlooked method of reducing noise exposure: silence. This is especially helpful for anyone who listens to radio, music, or television for long periods of time. Most of us have gotten so accustomed to having some kind of noise in the background that we forget it is often a choice. Simply turning off the news, music players, or programs you're not watching can give your ears a vacation from the constant assault by sound.

Another way to rest your ears is by seeking out quiet places. I have suggested this to a number of patients, with great success. This kind of "auditory vacation" is especially helpful for young people, who have grown up with nonstop sounds produced by everything from toys to technology. For example, I met Andy after three days at a music festival had left him with ringing ears, a condition known as tinnitus (see Chapter Twelve). When he described his typical day, it was clear that the festival wasn't the only reason for his tinnitus. Andy spent most of the day listening to his personal music player, rode a motorcycle without ear protection, and played video games with the volume on the highest setting.

I explained to Andy that we could get the tinnitus under control, but if he didn't eliminate some of the noise in his life, the condition could become permanent. The ringing in his ears was severe enough to motivate Andy, and he changed his ways. With the tinnitus remedy I recommended, plus earplugs, lower-volume entertainment, and "noise breaks" to rest his ears, Andy was much improved before long. He was also surprised that he didn't mind silence as much as he thought he would. "I really had a hard time with the idea of turning off my music and listening to *nothing*," he told me. "But now I kind of like it. I grab some lunch and go to the park to just relax and listen to as little as possible."

Keep in mind that people of all ages can benefit from noise breaks. Giving your ears a chance to rest and repair really can make a difference in hearing.

The Color of Noise

By now, you may be wondering exactly what "white noise" is and how sound can have color. Actually, the color is simply a label to define varying frequency characteristics. In technical terms, when a signal has a flat frequency spectrum, it is called white noise. In practice, it sounds a bit like a soft whooshing sound or that faint whisper of the ocean that can be heard in seashells.

White noise is considered soothing and a good way to block bothersome background noise. Fortunately, you can buy white-noise CDs that simulate a wide range of soothing sounds, including rainfall, waves on a shore, and a gentle breeze. (Technically speaking, these are not true white noise, but they do mask environmental noise quite well.) There are also white-noise CDs tailored to block specific annoying sounds. A "distant thunderstorm" version, for example, counteracts snoring and the thumping bass of boom boxes.

You can achieve the same end result—and more—with some of the devices now available that produce white noise designed not only to mask noise pollution but also to reduce the possibility of eavesdropping. Most of these "sound conditioners" are quite portable, and there are also travel models small enough to pack into a suitcase. If you've ever spent the night in a hotel near the airport or close to major transportation, you'll understand why the travel models are popular.

Many people report success in minimizing noise with these devices, including parents of infants and young children. In fact, there are scores of white-noise CDs designed specifically for families. While some of them border on the silly— mimicking sounds of vacuum cleaners, hair dryers, and the like—the parent of a colicky baby is very likely willing to try just about anything.

White noise can help adults sleep, too. Scientists at the National Center for Post-Traumatic Stress Disorder in Honolulu found white noise to be a simple, safe, inexpensive alternative to sleeping pills, useful for treating insomnia and post-traumatic stress disorder.[1]

Another hue—"pink" noise, which is essentially like white noise but with a bit of a rumble added in—has been helpful for individuals with hyperacusis, a disorder involving extraordinary sound sensitivity that makes everyday noise levels intolerable. There are other "colors" of noise—including brown, blue, purple, and gray—but discussing these gets into some fairly technical issues. Since white noise is the most pertinent to the subject of hearing and sound, we'll leave it at that.

Measuring Sound with a Meter

If you'd like to find out just how noisy your workplace—or your neighbor's stereo—is, you can use a *sound level meter* (SLM). These are typically handheld devices that can be used to measure decibel levels in most settings. SLMs tend to be pricey, easily costing several hundred dollars. But they can be a good investment for anyone who wants or needs to monitor sound levels, such as a business owner interested in protecting employees' hearing or meeting OSHA (Occupational Safety and Health Administration) standards. There are various types of SLMs, equipped with a wide range of features. Some SLMs, for example, come with an alarm (in the form of a large LCD that can be read from a distance, rather than yet another noise) that signals when sound levels go above a specific limit.

A *noise dosimeter* measures sound levels, too, but it's designed to be worn by an individual to monitor the amount of noise the person is being exposed to. Dosimeters are equipped with small microphones that are placed near the ears, to actually record noise levels the individual is hearing. These devices also measure the wearer's "noise dose calculations," so people working under noisy conditions can monitor sound levels that are reaching the ears and (hopefully) prevent hearing damage.

There are many other mechanisms for measuring noise pollution and environmental noise, both indoors and out. If noise is a problem and it needs to be measured and documented, there is probably a device designed to do that. A word of caution: Most of this equipment is fairly complex, so research the field before making a purchase, or talk to a sound expert about measuring sound levels for you.

Protecting Ears in the Air

Changes in atmospheric pressure while flying can have a significant effect on ears. Anyone who has flown while suffering with a cold has probably experienced the sharp pains caused by changes in cabin pressure. But the ears can suffer during flight even without congestion, especially during landings, when cabin pressure can escalate to uncomfortable levels. You can relieve some of this pressure by chewing gum during landings. For small children, the same net effect can be obtained by giving them a bottle of juice, milk, or water during takeoff and landing.

Over-the-counter decongestants, such as Sudafed, can also minimize the effects of atmospheric change while flying. The downside, though, is that decongestants are dehydrating. Combining these drugs with the low humidity found in airplane cabins can rob the body of necessary fluids, so drink plenty of water or juices before, during, and after the flight. Coffee, tea, and alcohol are not nearly as beneficial, since they tend to have a diuretic effect.

QUIETING THE BARKING DOG

Even the most devout dog lover can be annoyed by out-of-control barking. Whether it's your own pet or a neighbor's, there are alternatives to living with this problem. First, recognize that barking is perfectly normal behavior for dogs, and there is no method that can completely eliminate it. Even dogs that have been "debarked" by having tissue removed from the larynx still make an irritating coughing sound when they attempt to bark. In addition, the surgery only provides temporary results, because the tissue grows back.

If your own pet is barking excessively, consult a trainer or invest in a book or video that explains various humane methods of training a dog to bark less frequently. And remember that shouting at the dog is not only ineffective but adds to the noise. If the problem pooch belongs to a neighbor, however, be aware that many people consider pets to be family members, and criticism is likely to be unwelcome. Approach your neighbor in a friendly manner, and you're likely to get a better response than threatening to call Animal Control. Many people who work are not aware that their dog is barking, but attitude is everything when discussing this problem with a dog owner.

There are a number of training aids that can be useful when working with your own dog or dealing with a neighbor's. Ultrasonic training devices, for example, emit a high-frequency sound that can be heard only by dogs (and cats). Most dogs do not like the sound and stop barking when they hear it. These devices come in a variety of forms. The type that can be set up in the yard has one drawback: Users have noted that any loud noise occurring outside (such as a car horn, slamming door, or loud engine) can set it off, so the dog is likely to become confused. Portable models do not have this problem, because they are equipped with a button that must be pushed to activate the ultrasonic sound. This type of device can be attached to a belt or arm with a wrist strap, making them useful for other training purposes. For example, if your dog pulls or lunges while walking, sounding the trainer tells the dog that this behavior is unacceptable. Other options include "no bark" training collars that come equipped with either an ultrasonic device or citronella sprays that go off when barking occurs. (See pages 235 and 236 in Resources.)

The Sounds of Silence and the Science of Acoustics

Soundproofing wasn't the highest priority when Drew and Yukari were making plans to remodel their home. But when they decided that the best place for a media room was next to the master bedroom, they asked the architect what could be done to minimize sound leakage. "We realized that installing a media room and then expecting our kids to keep the volume down so we could have some peace and quiet was not going to work," Yukari explains. "So we had to look at ways to keep the sound inside the room."

They discovered there are plenty of options, depending largely on budget. Since the remodel was extensive, sound-baffling insulation, double-paned windows, and solid doors were obvious choices. In addition, they chose sound-absorbing fabric for the walls and ceilings and gained additional soundproofing by adding thick acoustical tiles to the wall between the media room and their bedroom. The couple also learned that using fabric throughout their bedroom would help muffle sounds. Double-lined, floor-length drapes, thick rugs with heavy pads underneath, and upholstered walls work together to keep the bedroom peaceful, even while the media room is filled with kids.

As you can see, ear protection choices run the gamut. Whatever your particular need may be, there is something that can shield your ears from the noise that is part of modern life. Even a low-cost option, like disposable foam earplugs, is better than nothing. But I encourage you to explore more sophisticated ear protection, because cutting down on noise in your environment really can make a difference.

((**10**))

PUTTING IT ALL TOGETHER: THE SAVE YOUR HEARING NOW PROGRAM IN ACTION

You've read all the advice and recommendations. You are ready to start making the lifestyle changes that are the cornerstones of the Save Your Hearing Now Program. Now what? A good place to begin is by recording some observations about your typical day. Write down what time you get up, what you have for breakfast, how long it takes to get to work, what you do during your breaks, what you eat for lunch and dinner, what you do after work, and what time you go to bed. Once you have this information, you can start making changes.

A little later in this chapter is a schedule for a typical Save Your Hearing Now day, including menu ideas and times for working out. You can compare your own day to this chart and see where improvements can be made.

Let's say, for example, that you get up at 7 a.m., shower, get dressed, and go to work. Right away, when you compare your morning to the chart, you will see that breakfast is missing. (If you need to be reminded about why breakfast is important, reread Chapter Seven.) Maybe getting up ten minutes earlier is all it takes to change that. If breakfast was not important, it would not be on the chart, so adjust your schedule accordingly.

Continue to compare what you are doing to the Save Your Hearing Now recommendations and see where improvements can be made. Remember, however, that the program is based on suggestions, not rules etched in stone. The program is designed to give you a chance to play an active role in your own health care management. And that involves learning to make good choices that are *appropriate for you.* The purpose of the chart is simply to illustrate one way of putting the Save Your Hearing Now principles to work. I encourage each individual to adapt it, as necessary, without eliminating any elements.

So, for example, although physical activity is divided into three sessions throughout the day, it may make more sense for you to accomplish the same goal with one workout, which is fine. On the other hand, some people may need to divvy up the total goal of sixty minutes per day into four or five sessions. Again, this is not a problem. Skipping the exercise component entirely, however, is not recommended (unless, of course, your physician has instructed you to do so or you do not have a doctor's permission to begin working out).

One more consideration: In the enthusiasm of beginning a new lifestyle plan, many people go overboard and try to change everything at once. Sometimes this works, but it can also be overwhelming. If you choose to go "cold turkey" and leave all your old habits behind, please don't become frustrated with your progress—or lack of it—and throw in the towel. Whatever you are hoping to improve—whether it's hearing, weight, or fitness—remember that it most likely required years for you to get to this point. It is simply not possible to reverse the accumulated damage in a couple of weeks or even months. Commit to making these changes for the long haul, not as a temporary, quick fix.

Lifestyle Chart

On the chart below, you can record information about your typical day. Compare it to the Save Your Hearing Now daily plan on page 188 to find ways to incorporate the recommended lifestyle changes. Note the following:

What time did you get up?

What time did you eat each meal and snack, and what did you eat? Include beverages as well as food.

What time did you take any nutritional supplements, and what did you take?

What time did you exercise, and for how long?

What did you do in the evening, and how much time did you spend on each activity? (For those who work in the evening or night shift, note what you did after work and for how long.)

What time did you go to sleep?

---

6 a.m.

---

7 a.m.

---

8 a.m.

9 a.m.

10 a.m.

11 a.m.

Noon

1 p.m.

2 p.m.

3 p.m.

4 p.m.

5 p.m.

6 p.m.

7 p.m.

8 p.m.

9 p.m.

10 p.m.

11 p.m.

Midnight

1 a.m.

2 a.m.

3 a.m.

4 a.m.

5 a.m.

Change is difficult for many people. If you find yourself resisting some element of the program, stop and think about why that is happening. Do you absolutely hate brown rice? Or is the real problem that you had a tough day at work and long for the comforting taste of a baked potato stuffed with sour cream, butter, and chives? If that is the correct answer, keep this in mind: The brown rice is loaded with B vitamins that can take the edge off stress, while the baked potato is loaded with . . . well, sour cream and butter, which are mostly saturated fat. Sure, the potato will taste good, but what about the guilt that will follow, not to mention the high-calorie, artery-clogging fat your body has to cope with? Start thinking of the body as a machine, like a well-designed car. Put the right fuel (food) into it and maintain it (exercise) appropriately, and it will perform with far more efficiency than if you fill the tank with potato chips and dip and let it sit in the garage for weeks on end. If the human body came with an owner's manual, it would be very similar to the Save Your Hearing Now Program.

A Typical Day on the Save Your Hearing Now Program

Compare your own typical day with the recommendations below to see where you can make lifestyle changes to support good hearing. Certain recommendations, such as the time you choose to engage in physical activity, are flexible. However, I highly encourage you not to eliminate any elements, unless your physician has advised you to do so. Although this chart does not include the standard recommendation for eight glasses of water each day, please aim for that amount every day.

  Note: Many of the food choices listed here are part of a Mediterranean-style eating plan, because the Mediterranean diet has repeatedly been shown to be a good-for-the-heart plan that incorporates abundant amounts of fruits, vegetables, and good fats, as well as great flavor and variety. There are a number of cookbooks focusing on this diet, so you should have no trouble finding recipes.

7 a.m.   **Breakfast:** Scrambled eggs or egg substitute with one-half cup spinach, a few pine nuts, and a sprinkle of grated hard cheese like Romano or Pecorino. Whole-wheat toast with cholesterol-lowering spread containing plant sterols (available in most supermarkets). Small orange or glass of orange juice, preferably with pulp (for fiber!). Coffee or tea.

Supplements: Take half of the recommended dosage of the Save Your Hearing Now Top Ten supplements (ALA, ALC, vitamin B complex, CoQ10, glutathione, lecithin, NAC, quercetin, resveratrol, and zinc) after breakfast, along with your daily multivitamin/mineral and the additional supporting supplements. Drink at least eight ounces of water with the supplements. If you are taking other medications, it is best to take nutritional supplements two to three hours before or after the prescription medications.

Activity: Twenty-minute walk with two minutes of easy stretching before and after. Take along a bottle of water.

---

10 a.m. **Midmorning snack:** Small box of raisins, a handful of baby carrots, one-quarter cup no-salt peanuts.

---

1 p.m.   **Lunch:** Grilled salmon (no more than four ounces, about the size of a deck of playing cards) on a bed of at least one cup salad greens, with cherry tomatoes, chickpeas, marinated artichoke hearts, and cucumber slices. For a dressing, mix one tablespoon olive or grape-seed oil with one teaspoon lemon juice and season with herbs and pepper to taste. Whole-wheat roll with small amount (one tablespoon) of olive oil for dipping. Tea or water with a slice of citrus. For dessert, one-half cup red grapes.

Supplements: Take the second half of the daily supplement dosage after lunch, if possible, or following the evening meal, with at least eight ounces of water. Also take additional supporting supplements as necessary to reach the recommended daily dosage. Example: If your multivitamin supplies less than 100 mg of vitamin C, you won't be getting the Save Your Hearing Now recommended dosage of 100 to 1,500 mg from the multi alone. If that's the case, add extra C at lunch or dinner, or possibly even both. As a water-soluble nutrient, this much-needed antioxidant needs to be constantly replenished in the body.

Activity: Ten-minute walk (or longer) after lunch.

---

4 p.m. **Midday snack:** Fresh or canned (without added sugar) pear and one-ounce portion of reduced-fat cheese. The combination of complex carbohydrates in the pear and protein in the cheese can supply the energy to get through the typical afternoon slump. Tea (decaf so sleep is not affected) or more water, or both.

---

7 p.m. **Dinner:** Brown rice pilaf with white beans and oregano seasoning. Shish kebab consisting of mostly veggies (onions, tomatoes, peppers, zucchini) and no more than four ounces protein (chicken, fish, tofu). Grilled or broiled asparagus, lightly seasoned with grape-seed or canola oil and favorite seasonings. Whole-wheat roll with one tablespoon olive oil. If you're in the mood for something sweet for dessert, try a baked apple seasoned with cinnamon and nutmeg, topped with one-half cup berries and a spritz of

reduced-fat whipping cream. Glass of red wine (optional) or grape or pomegranate juice.

Supplements: If you have not reached the recommended levels of nutrients on the Save Your Hearing Now Program, this is the time to take additional doses.

Activity: Before or after dinner, spend an additional twenty minutes walking or doing another type of aerobic activity, plus a few minutes of stretching before and after.

---

9 p.m.   **Evening snack:** Two cups of air-popped popcorn with small amount of butter-flavored spray.

---

11 p.m. **Bedtime.**

((11))

SO LONG, STRESS, AND GOOD-BYE, BLUES!

Like most chronic health concerns, hearing loss has emotional consequences. Stress and depression are two of the most common. Robbed of the very basic and important ability to communicate, individuals with hearing loss often feel cut off from family, friends, and much of the world. Social settings, both recreational and work-related, become stressful when hearing is difficult. The alternative, however, is to spend time alone, and for many people, depression goes hand in hand with loneliness.

The stress involved in living with hearing loss can be minimized. Similarly, if depression is an issue, it should be treated. Ignoring either one simply won't work. Both can have a profound impact on health. But scientists are learning that there is a great deal we can do to protect ourselves.

The Stress Factor

Stress is an unavoidable part of life. For years, we've been told stress is bad, but the truth is human beings are designed to benefit from stress. Surges of stress hormones like adrenaline and cortisol helped early humans stay alive in a dangerous world. Today, our environment is more civilized, but those same hormones enable us to embark on risky ventures, like attempting to surf an oncoming wave, enter the traffic stream on a busy freeway, or ask the boss for a day off. And let's not forget about the good side of stress, or "eustress," that makes some of life's most exciting moments—landing a new job, getting married, having a baby—so unforgettable.

Clearly, we cannot escape stress completely. But we should learn to manage the negative form—"distress"—effectively, because it has been linked to a long list of health problems. Among them: heart disease, diabetes, obesity, accelerated aging, and depression. As we have seen, all these conditions can contribute to hearing loss. In addition, because stress constricts the blood vessels throughout the body, the cochlea's hair cells—along with all the body's cells—are deprived of the oxygen they need to thrive. Clearly, minimizing stress is an excellent method of protecting hearing and much more.

To understand how stress compromises health, let's look at some recent scientific discoveries. One revealing example of the downside of stress—as well as a means of coping with it—was discovered by scientists at the University of California, San Francisco. They found that women who live with long-term stress actually age faster at the cellular level. Researchers examined blood cells from women who were caring for children with chronic disabilities and compared those cells to others taken from a group of women who were not caregivers. Significant age-related cell damage was found among women in the first group. In fact, cells from some women in the high-stress group showed signs of aging that were ten years or more beyond their actual age.

There was a second finding in this study, however, and one that is very important to remember. Researchers found that the caregiving women who did not perceive their situation as stressful were not affected at the cellular level.[1] In other words, stress is in the eye of the beholder. An individual who considers a demanding job to be a wonderful opportunity, for example, is not going to suffer the same negative effects as a co-worker who feels trapped and desperate. The bottom line: Change a potentially damaging stressful situation by changing your perspective.

Minimizing Stress with Food and Supplements

Clearly, stress can be reduced by a change in attitude. One way to support that change is by "feeding" the brain mood-enhancing nutrients, like complex carbohydrates. According to a recent review of studies focusing on stress and nutrition, increasing levels of the amino acid tryptophan in the brain with a diet high in complex carbs and low in protein encourages production of serotonin, a feel-good brain chemical. The complex carbohydrates that are part of the Save Your Hearing Now Program—whole grains, vegetables, and fruits—are far more healthful than simple carbs found in sugar and processed foods. In addition to supplying serotonin's building blocks, complex carbs also provide healthy doses of fiber, antioxidants, and other nutrients, like stress-combating B vitamins.

The essential fatty acids known as the omega-3s (see Chapter Six) have been shown in clinical trials to tame what researchers call stress-induced aggression and hostility. Furthermore, a study of adults in stressful positions found that a daily dose of 6 grams of fish oil, containing 1.5 grams of docosahexaenoic acid (DHA), resulted in significant reductions in the perceptions of stress.[2]

Some Simple Stress Reduction Techniques

No news is good news. British researchers found that watching as little as fifteen minutes of news on an average day left viewers feeling confused, angry, anxious, depressed, and irritated. Comedy is a much better destressor. Studies have shown that laughter increases levels of feel-good chemicals in the brain.

Get a pet. A growing body of research shows that pet owners are considerably healthier than those without an animal companion in some important ways, including diminished stress levels. And if you need to get active, having a dog to walk is a great way to get going.

Take time for you. Even short sessions of meditation have repeatedly been shown to have profound benefits when it comes to stress reduction and renewed mental functions. Even something as simple as envisioning a stressful event with a positive outcome can be helpful.

Spend some time with Mozart. At Roosevelt University Stress Institute in Chicago, researchers compared the effects of three different twenty-eight-minute breaks on a group of volunteers. One group listened to recordings of Mozart's work, another was entertained with New Age music, and the third spent their time reading magazines. After only three days, members of the Mozart group had the lowest stress levels and reported the greatest feelings of relaxation.[3]

Stay social. Hearing loss can make socializing difficult. But instead of turning to solitary pursuits, simply tell friends that you're having some trouble with hearing and ask that they speak up. No one apologizes for wearing glasses. Why should hearing loss be any different than correcting eyesight?

Share your situation. Tell the people around you that you're making changes to improve your hearing. Few things are more stressful than trying to keep a secret.

Connect on the Internet. There are dozens of sites on the Internet where individuals with hearing loss can gather information and exchange stories. Using the Internet allows social opportunities that don't strain listening abilities. The Resources section lists some good places to start.

Recognize that men and women are different. When it comes to coping with stress, men tend to turn to sports and other distractions that help them forget the situation. Women, on the other hand, prefer communication and are more likely to talk about the stresses they experience. There is no right or wrong here. Whatever works is fine.

Write about it. Several studies have found that people who simply write down what is bothering them and how they feel about it have lower levels of stress hormones than those who were not instructed to write about their experiences. Don't feel that your writing has to be grammatical, poetic, or even make sense. The point is to relay inner emotions to an outside source.

EXERCISING AWAY STRESS

Rosa got the bad news during a physical examination when she was applying for new health insurance. Her blood pressure was far too high, and she weighed about sixty pounds too much. "I had been dieting like crazy most of my life," she recalls. "But I manage a restaurant, and every day the chefs make something new that we have to try."

The good news was that the food Rosa was eating was

high-quality and prepared by an exceptional team of professionals. The bad news was that she was eating far too much of it. "The job stress in the restaurant business is off the charts," she explained. "Customers are demanding, chefs can be temperamental, the suppliers drop the ball, and you end up with food you can't use for one reason or another. Between trying to keep costs down and make everyone happy, I was a basket case. So I ate."

Rosa's doctor thoroughly explained the dangers of excess weight and how they are compounded by lack of exercise and a high-stress job. Because her aunt and an older sister both had breast cancer, Rosa was already motivated to change her lifestyle, so her doctor referred her to a nutritionist, who helped her come up with a plan.

Since Rosa couldn't escape food—"How can I recommend something to customers if I haven't tried it?"— her nutritionist suggested she promise herself not to eat more than one or two bites of the new dishes that were being tested every day. The guilt of overeating on a daily basis was one profound source of stress that Rosa could eliminate.

She also met with a personal trainer and followed his advice to wear a pedometer. "Right away, I saw that even though I was on my feet most of the day, I wasn't *moving*," she said. "Even when I started taking little walking breaks, I wasn't even close to the 10,000-steps-per-day goal."

To change that, Rosa started setting aside thirty to sixty minutes each evening for the treadmill. At first, she resented every minute of it. There were so many other things she could be doing with that time! But then it dawned on her: Why not multitask on the treadmill, just like she did at work? Rosa bought a stack of books on tape and began working her way through all the reading she had been postponing. After about two weeks, Rosa was happily surprised to find that her clothes were much looser and she had more energy. Plus, she was catching up on her reading. "But it was the effect exercise had on my stress levels that really convinced me to keep going," she explained. "My blood pressure is nearly normal now, and I don't feel like I'm going to blow a gasket when the inevitable problems come up at work. My only regret is that I didn't start doing this a long time ago."

Dealing with Depression

Some 20 million Americans live with depression, according to the National Institute of Mental Health, and twice as many women as men are affected by the disease. Combine the cost of various forms of treatment with lost productivity in the workplace, and the figure tops $40 billion annually. Obviously, depression costs society dearly, but it takes a personal toll, too, causing friction in a marriage or family and affecting an individual's performance in the workplace. Health suffers as well. Depression has been linked to immune disorders, heart disease, diabetes, and a host of other complications. At the most severe end of the spectrum, depression can be so overwhelming that each year thousands of people in this country choose to end their lives, including a number of elderly individuals.

Depression is difficult to diagnose and can be challenging to treat. Based on a recent survey, the National Depressive and Manic Depressive Association determined that more than half of all people suffering from depression are not properly diagnosed or treated by their physicians. In part, this is no doubt due to the fact that symptoms run the gamut and vary considerably from one person to another. Insomnia, for example, can be caused by depression, but so can excessive sleeping. Fatigue, digestive disorders, back pain, headaches, loss or increase in appetite, mood swings, feelings of worthlessness, inability to concentrate, and avoidance of social situations may also occur.

Although depression is an emotional issue, it has physical consequences. For example, a team of scientists at Emory University and Yale University found that depression can damage the heart. Fifty pairs of healthy, middle-aged male twins were monitored by electrocardiograms for twenty-four hours. During that time, researchers also conducted tests to measure depression levels among participants. In the end, they discovered a link between depression and reduced heart rate variability (HRV), a measure of fluctuations between heartbeats. A decrease in HRV can make the heart susceptible to arrhythmias and sudden fatalities.[4]

The Elderly Are More Vulnerable to Depression

Depression can happen to anyone, at any age. But it is particularly common among the elderly and is frequently partnered with hearing loss and social isolation. As Helen Keller observed, living with blindness was difficult, but losing the ability to hear was worse. "When you lose your vision you lose contact with things," she explained. "When you lose your hearing you lose contact with people."

A study conducted by the National Council on the Aging summed up the situation this way: Untreated hearing loss frequently results in social isolation, which in turn contributes to depression, anxiety, and/or paranoia. Unfortunately, depression is already common among older people, regardless of their hearing abilities. About half of all seniors living in nursing homes may be suffering from depression, according to the American Psychological Association, along with approximately 20 percent of the seniors who are living on their own.

Are antidepressants the answer? A recent report from the U.S. Department of Health and Human Services shows that antidepressants are hugely popular in this country, with nearly triple the number of prescriptions being written today as there were just ten years ago. Unfortunately, those drugs may not be doing the job. According to the results of a recent survey, based on querying some twelve hundred patients being treated for depression with a combination of antidepressants and therapy, researchers determined that about half of those individuals did not experience any improvement.

Ineffectiveness is not the only problem linked to antidepressants, though. Several other studies have found serious side effects associated with popular antidepressant medications, such as the selective serotonin reuptake inhibitors (SSRIs), a group that includes the popular Prozac. One group of medical experts found a significant increase in bone loss among postmenopausal women on SSRIs, while an animal study showed that young animals given antidepressants had smaller, weaker bones in adulthood than those that did not receive the medications.[5] Furthermore, a third study from the Netherlands reported an increase in abnormal bleeding in patients taking SSRIs.[6]

A Better Way to Deal with Depression

Of course, depression should be treated with the help of a qualified physician or therapist. Fortunately, alternative medicine offers a number of effective remedies for mild to moderate depression, including the omega-3 essential fatty acids, vitamin D, the herb St.-John's-wort, and the amino acid *S*-adenosyl-methionine (SAM-e). But even these remedies might not be necessary for individuals who are willing to invest some time in physical activity. Talk with your doctor about all the available conventional and alternative approaches to treating depression and which is best for you.

Researchers at the University of Georgia, for example,

found that an increase in physical activity reduces symptoms of depression in youngsters.[7] In addition, the results of a new study from the University of Texas Southwestern Medical Center show that adults between the ages of twenty and forty-five with mild to moderate depression experienced a fifty percent improvement in symptoms if they took part in half an hour of sustained aerobic exercise three to five times per week.[8] Furthermore, researchers at Duke University found that regular moderate exercise was just as effective as the prescription antidepressant Zoloft for treating major depression.[9] In my opinion, this is a real milestone. The side effects of pharmaceutical antidepressants, like Zoloft and Prozac, are a problem for many people. But this study shows that even those with serious depression can get relief from brisk workouts three times a week in thirty-minute sessions.

Finally, after reviewing more than thirty studies focusing on mood and activity levels in older people, researchers at Arizona State University determined that both aerobic and strength-training exercises were effective at improving mood. In fact, low-intensity workouts were the best mood boosters of all.[10]

CAN A HEARING TEST DETERMINE ANTIDEPRESSANT EFFECTIVENESS?

Fascinating results from preliminary research at Columbia University show that depression, hearing, and medication effectiveness may be interrelated, at least in women. Typically, doctors use a trial and error method to find an appropriate remedy. If a patient does not respond to one antidepressant, the doctor will recommend another and so on, in hopes of finding one that works. But in three separate studies, the experts at Columbia discovered that a very basic listening test can help determine which female patients benefit from the class of antidepressants known as SSRIs (selective serotonin reuptake inhibitors).

Researchers tested hearing in a group of women, half of whom were depressed. The simple test required the women to wear headphones while two words were read at the same time. The women with depression who identified the words most clearly turned out to be the same ones who responded successfully to SSRIs. Experts are not certain why or how hearing and depression are connected, although they speculate that imbalances in left- and right-brain activity play a role.

The results of the initial study have been replicated twice. Based on this research, the scientists have found that women with depression who respond with above-average hearing (i.e., left-brain activity) also have a 95 percent success rate with Prozac. Of course, this approach still needs further study before it is likely to turn up in physicians' offices. But it does offer hope that one day soon it may be possible to apply these lessons and refine the prescribing of antidepressants.[11]

The Right Fats Fight Depression

Thirty years ago, all fat was declared a health hazard. Today, after hundreds of studies examining various aspects of fat, experts realize that fats cannot be lumped into one category. Some should be avoided (saturated and trans fats, for example). Meanwhile, intake of others, like the "good" omega-3s, need to be increased, either by adding more fish or flax to the diet or via supplements. At the same time, consumption of omega-6s, the vegetable oils found in snacks, chips, and many processed foods, should be reduced. The goal is to reach a better ratio, such as 3:1, in regard to omega-3s and omega-6s than the current 1:20.

Within the omega-3 category, as we saw in Chapter Seven, there are three different types of fats: alpha-linolenic acid (ALA), docosahexaenoic acid (DHA), and eicosapentaenoic acid (EPA). Fatty types of fish—salmon, sardines, cod, tuna, halibut, mackerel, sea bass, and anchovies—are rich in DHA and EPA. Flaxseeds or flax oil is the best source of ALA, but canola oil, hemp seeds, walnuts, and wheat germ, as well as their oils, also supply this nutrient. The omega-3s offer impressive overall health benefits, and that includes easing symptoms of depression.[12]

Shining New Light on Vitamin D

For years, we were told that a little vitamin D goes a long way. Respected medical experts warned of toxic effects at high doses, and while other nutrients stole the limelight, vitamin D remained quietly in the background.

Now, as we discussed in Chapter Six, the story on vitamin D has changed. Dozens of new studies show that vitamin D is a rising superstar in the health arena. Not only is it linked to hearing, but it also helps keep bones strong and healthy and protects against heart disease, high blood pressure, cancer, and depression.

Unfortunately, some experts believe that vitamin D deficiencies are widespread, primarily due to warnings to stay out of the sun (under proper conditions, the body produces vitamin D with small amounts of sun exposure). People who followed that advice and regularly avoided the sun are among those most likely to be lacking in vitamin D. In addition, people with dark skin, housebound individuals, and anyone living in a cold, northern climate are also at risk for deficiencies. Add to this the fact that few foods provide vitamin D (some types of seafood, such as mackerel, herring, and salmon, eggs, and fortified milk and dairy products are the best sources), and it's easy to see how deficiencies can occur.

Research from the University of Toronto shows that vitamin D supplements can ease symptoms of depression. The study involved 130 patients suffering from depression who all had normal blood levels of vitamin D. The group was divided into two portions. One group was given a minimal daily dose of 600 IU of vitamin D_3 (also known as cholecalciferol), while the other was treated with 4,000 IU of vitamin D_3, an amount many experts believe to be far more appropriate for therapeutic purposes. After following this regimen for one year, researchers found that levels of depression had improved in both groups, but those who were given 4,000 IU benefited most.[13]

Recommendations for daily intake of vitamin D have recently been revised. Instead of an RDA, the federal government now recommends that adult men and women up to age fifty take 200 IU per day. Between ages fifty-one and seventy, the recommended amount is 400 IU daily, and after seventy-one, it is 600 IU. Since vitamin D is fat-soluble and therefore can accumulate in the body, megadoses (more than 65,000 IU daily) are not recommended.

If you prefer to make your own vitamin D, here's the "recipe" for a light-skinned (Caucasian) individual: Expose bare skin on the arms to sunlight for fifteen to twenty minutes three to five days each week. This will produce about 10,000 IU of vitamin D, the equivalent of what is typically found in twenty-five multivitamins or one hundred glasses of fortified milk. Spending more time in the sun does not increase production—the body seems to have an established production quota, so you cannot overdose on sunlight-created vitamin D—but extra sun exposure could increase the risk of developing skin cancer.

Chasing the Blues Away with St.-John's-Wort

The herb known as St.-John's-wort is a common perennial found throughout Europe and North America. It has been used for centuries to treat wounds, as well as relieve anxiety, stress, and depression. In recent years, conflicting findings from studies have cast doubt on the effectiveness of St.-John's-wort as a remedy for depression. But two new clinical trials support the herb's effectiveness. Both were conducted in Germany, and both compared the effects of the herbal remedy with either Zoloft or Paxil, two very popular prescription antidepressants. In each case, St.-John's-wort was at least as effective as the prescription drug and was associated with fewer side effects.[14]

Talk with your doctor about which brand and dosage might be best for you, then look for a product containing a standardized *Hypericum* (the active ingredient) extract. (Just for the record, in one of the two German studies, the dosage used was 612 mg of *Hypericum* extract given once daily, while the other used 300 mg supplements taken three times a day.)

Get to Know SAM-e

SAM-e (*S*-adenosyl-methionine) is an amino acid used by the body in dozens of processes, including the manufacture of DNA and mood-regulating neurotransmitters, such as dopamine. SAM-e also serves as an antioxidant, helps maintain healthy cells, and protects the tissues in the joints. A number of studies have also shown that SAM-e can ease symptoms of depression. While it may take as long as six weeks of steady intake for St.-John's-wort to reach maximum effectiveness, SAM-e often provides much more rapid relief.

Furthermore, SAM-e appears to have the unique ability to boost the effectiveness of prescription antidepressants. Researchers at Harvard Medical School reported nearly 100 percent success in treating depression with prescription medication in conjunction with SAM-e. The combination was tested in a group of depression sufferers who did not benefit from prescription antidepressants alone. When SAM-e was added to their regimen, however, 50 percent of the participants had improvement in depression symptoms after six weeks, and 43 percent said they no longer felt depressed at all.[15]

The typical prescribed dosage of SAM-e is 400 mg daily, but up to 800 mg daily is sometimes used to treat depression. If mild nausea occurs, talk to your doctor about trying a different SAM-e product, as not all produce this side effect.

Here are a few other suggestions to ease feelings of depression:

Sit up straight. Canadian researchers found that when people sit in an upright position, it is more than 90 percent easier to generate positive thoughts than while sitting slumped over.[16]

Try yoga. After practicing yoga for five months, a group of men and women had fewer symptoms of anxiety and depression, as well as better flexibility and improved mental abilities, when compared with a sedentary control group.[17]

Have a checkup. Depression can be a symptom of vitamin deficiency, allergy (including food allergy or sensitivity), or thyroid problems. A thorough physical can help identify the cause.

Are you depressed, or is it SAD? Seasonal affective disorder (SAD) occurs during the short days of winter when sunlight is reduced. SAD can be treated by installing full-spectrum lightbulbs in the workplace and at home. There are also special light boxes available to treat this disorder. A natural health-care practitioner can recommend an appropriate model.

((12))

LISTENING TO MOTHER NATURE: ALTERNATIVE REMEDIES FOR OTHER HEARING PROBLEMS

Tinnitus

"The buzzing in my ears was driving me crazy."

Four years ago, Jean-Paul, a commercial artist, went into the hospital for a hernia operation. A reaction to the anesthesia he was given left him feeling wired. "It just shattered my nerves," he recalls.

The family doctor prescribed medicine that made him feel calm during the day but left him restless and unable to sleep at night. A second prescription for sleep medication was only partially successful. Jean-Paul dozed off but then woke up six to eight times each night. After eight months without a decent night's sleep, he retuned to the doctor and was given Zoloft. Soon after he started taking the antidepressant, his ears began buzzing.

The buzzing itself wasn't unusual; ever since he was in his twenties, Jean-Paul had dealt with sporadic "buzzing episodes," the result of accumulations of earwax that the doctor simply removed. But this time, cleaning his ears didn't

help. Jean-Paul stopped taking Zoloft, but the buzzing remained. "It was so loud it was making me nervous," he remembers. "The doctor told me I had tinnitus and there was
nothing he could do for me."

Some 35 million Americans live with tinnitus, and the
sounds they hear range from buzzing, like Jean-Paul, to
ringing, humming, hissing, clicking, roaring, whistling, and
whooshing. Exposure to loud noise can cause tinnitus, as can
certain medications. When the tinnitus sounds are not particularly loud, the condition is no more than a minor distrac-
tion. For Jean-Paul, that was not the case. "On a scale of one
to ten, with ten as insane, it was close to ten," he explains. "It
was really, really bad, and it was driving me crazy."

Frustrated by traditional medicine's inability to help him,
Jean-Paul began doing his own research. He discovered that
doctors in Europe frequently prescribe herbs for insomnia,
and he began using himself as a guinea pig. Eventually, Jean-
Paul found that a combination of valerian and hops enabled
him to sleep through the night.

Next, he decided to try the herb ginkgo biloba, which several studies had shown improved tinnitus symptoms by rebuilding blood vessels. The results were disappointing. Then
he came to see me. I suggested he increase the dosage of
ginkgo from 250 mg to 480 mg daily and take the antioxidants that are part of the Save Your Hearing Now Program.

Before long, Jean-Paul's tinnitus was under control. "It
didn't happen overnight, but pretty quickly the buzzing went
down to a level I can live with."

Ginkgo biloba has relieved tinnitus symptoms for many individuals, but not all. Just like prescription medications, alternative remedies, including herbs, do not work the same
way for everyone.[1] But if you are living with tinnitus, ginkgo
biloba is certainly worth discussing with your doctor and
trying, unless you are taking prescription blood thinners. In
addition, nearly all the supplements recommended as part of

the Save Your Hearing Now Program are also helpful for reducing tinnitus symptoms, particularly the mineral zinc. Furthermore, a garlic supplement (300 mg daily), which assists in blood pressure management, stress control, and minimizing cholesterol deposits that can block the small artery leading to the inner ear, can ease tinnitus symptoms. Although fresh garlic can be used in cooking, deodorized garlic supplements are useful for people who don't want to live with garlic's aftertaste.

The Mystery of Ménière's Disease

Tinnitus is sometimes involved in Ménière's disease, a multisymptom disorder that can include dizziness, hearing loss, nausea, fatigue, and a sensation of "stuffiness" in one ear or both. A relatively rare disorder, Ménière's disease is thought to be caused by excessive amounts of fluid (endolymph) in the semicircular canals of the inner ear. The fluid swells the membranes, disrupts hearing, and wreaks havoc with the sense of balance. No one yet knows why the fluid accumulates in the first place, although stress, autoimmune disease, a metabolic disorder, poor circulation, allergies, or a flawed gene are all possibilities. In fact, everything about Ménière's is a mystery. There is no real test for it, so it is generally diagnosed by ruling out everything else. Sometimes Ménière's occurs as a onetime experience, but it can also come and go, or simply arrive and stay.

Treating Ménière's is difficult, but if you are experiencing any of the symptoms, start with a visit to a physician to rule out other disorders. If a doctor suspects that Ménière's may be the cause of the problem, diuretics (water pills) and a low-salt diet are usually prescribed, aimed at reducing the amount of fluid in the ear. Caffeine, alcohol, and smoking are also prohibited. Alternative remedies include stress-fighting vitamin B complex, the mineral manganese, and CoQ10 to stimulate circulation.

Easing the Symptoms of Ear Infections

Few children grow up without experiencing at least one ear infection. The most common diagnosis is otitis media, or infection of the middle ear. In this case, the infection occurs behind the eardrum and can cause severe pain, fever, and a feeling of pressure in the ear, as well as difficulty hearing. Not so long ago, antibiotics were routinely prescribed to treat ear infections, but we now know that they were actually being overprescribed. This practice resulted in many children developing a tolerance to the antibiotics that rendered them ineffective. Today, doctors tend to hold off on the antibiotics unless the child has a high fever or other signs of infection. Ear infections generally improve in two to three days, without antibiotics. But there are other methods of reducing the pain and discomfort the child is experiencing.

Researchers in Israel, for example, conducted a clinical trial with more than 170 children suffering from ear infections with earaches to determine how a naturopathic remedy compared to antibiotic therapy. They found that naturopathic ear drops (consisting primarily of herbal extracts, plus vitamin E in olive oil, with or without a topical anesthetic to ease pain) were just as effective at reducing ear pain over a three-day period as antibiotics. The scientists also noted that the herbal extracts were easy to use, inexpensive compared to antibiotics, and had no side effects.[2]

A related study from Germany, comparing conventional ear-infection treatments with a highly diluted, plant-based remedy, had similar findings in a group of nearly four hundred youngsters between the ages of one and ten. Children who were given the alternative product experienced the same improvements as those receiving standard antibiotic care.[3]

If your child is experiencing ear infections, discuss antibiotic options with your pediatrician or ENT. Certainly, there are times when antibiotics are appropriate and even necessary. But for a simple ear infection, antibiotics are not always the best solution.

Alternative medicine has made great strides in terms of acceptance during the past twenty years, providing millions of individuals with relief for health conditions that conventional medicine cannot remedy, such as tinnitus. Of course, mainstream, traditional medicine certainly plays an important role in health. But increasingly, doctors are realizing that patients are interested in solutions regardless of the source.

It is important to keep in mind, however, that even though herbs and nutrients are natural, they sometimes have side effects in the same way as pharmaceutical drugs. In addition, there have been relatively few studies looking at alternative remedies and possible drug interactions. Anyone who is taking medication for a chronic ailment should always discuss adding herbs or other substances to the regimen. Conversely, if you are using nutritional supplements or alternative remedies and your physician recommends a prescription drug, be sure to tell her or him about the nutrients you are already taking.

((**13**))

HELP FROM HEARING AIDS

Like most chronic health conditions, hearing loss can be overwhelming and have heartbreaking consequences. But because there are no outward signs, many people try hard to compensate for hearing difficulties and pretend everything is fine. Yet inevitably, there comes a day when they can no longer deny there is a problem. Unfortunately, the obvious solution—a hearing aid—is not something most people embrace.

If hearing loss causes so many problems, why don't more people wear hearing aids? That question has several answers. First, there's the fact that the typical decline in hearing is so gradual that we unwittingly compensate for it for years. After all, at first, it's just a word missed here and there, and usually the context makes it clear.

Eventually, individuals experiencing hearing loss may find themselves unintentionally leaning this way or that, because hearing is usually sharper in one ear. Still, these little maneuvers are barely noticeable, more of a nuisance than a wake-up call. That usually arrives in the form of another person's comments. "Why is the TV always so loud?" a spouse or child may ask. Or a business associate might remark, "That was all explained in the meeting. Weren't you listening?" And even then, if the only alternative is a hearing aid, denial is very powerful. "Those are for geezers," said one fifty-something lawyer who admitted he had to strain to hear testimony in court. "What would my clients think if they saw me wearing a hearing aid?"

Second, although our ability to hear is essential for communication, many people don't—or won't—acknowledge difficulty hearing. One reason may be that coming to terms with hearing loss often means facing our own mortality. It's a sign not just of growing older but of deterioration, conjuring up images of frail, doddering old people with big, clumsy hearing aids perched on their ears. Because they are so closely associated with aging and decline, hearing aids carry a profound stigma.

As a result, the same person who wouldn't hesitate to wear glasses may refuse even to think about a hearing aid. Why the double standard? One theory is that our visually oriented culture makes us much more aware of—and likely to correct—failing eyesight. And glasses can be fashionable, even chic.

But hearing aids are in a completely different class. Compliments like "Nice hearing aid! Where did you get it?" are about as likely as a line of hearing devices created by a high-profile fashion designer. Neither one is going to happen because there's simply no way to make a skin-toned plastic blob look like a stylish accessory. Although there have been vast strides made in reducing the size and visibility of hearing devices, many people are so reluctant to discuss hearing aids that they aren't even aware of these improvements. As far as they're concerned, there's no socially acceptable remedy available, and so hearing loss goes untreated.

Another difference between glasses and hearing aids is that as soon as you put on a pair of glasses, vision becomes normal. But hearing aids can be very difficult to get used to because they amplify *all* sounds—not just the ones you want to hear. Normally, this problem can be overcome with repeat visits to the audiologist for adjustments, but many first-time hearing aid users are so disappointed by the initial experience that they simply refuse to wear them again.

HEARING "TOO MUCH"

Like many older individuals, Sam had to be coaxed and prodded into trying hearing aids. His initial impression— that he could hear "too much"—was a common reaction. After years of poor hearing, being confronted with a sudden amplification of sound is overwhelming. Like many people who don't want hearing aids in the first place, Sam simply refused to wear them. "We practically had to drag him kicking and screaming to the doctor to begin with," explained Sam's son. "And as soon as the hearing aids were in place, I could tell he was upset. By the time we got home twenty minutes later, he had already taken them off. He said he couldn't stand hearing so much. His exact words were, 'I will never wear those damn hearing aids again.'

"I begged him to have them adjusted, but there was just no way to get him to go back. So he had several thousand dollars' worth of equipment that could have helped him hear better sitting in a drawer, and never wore any of it again."

The Emotional Toll of Hearing Loss

In a fascinating series of studies conducted in 2000, hearing expert Sergei Kochkin discovered just how powerful the stigma of hearing loss—and resistance to hearing aids—can be. Although millions of Americans live with hearing impairment, Kochkin found that only one hearing-impaired individual in five has a hearing aid. And in the segment of the population between ages thirty-five and fifty-four, that figure dropped dramatically. In this group, Kochkin determined that 9 million individuals had hearing difficulties, yet a mere fraction—only 10 percent—used hearing aids.

Kochkin's findings are supported by a 1999 study from the National Council on the Aging (NCOA). According to that survey, among hearing-impaired Americans aged forty-five to sixty-four, only one in seven relied on a hearing aid. In the sixty-five and older age group the figure was slightly higher, with just two in five hearing-impaired individuals using hearing aids.

The NCOA survey also found that anxiety, depression, worry, emotional insecurity, social isolation, and paranoia were considerably more prevalent among hearing-impaired people over the age of fifty without hearing aids than in those who used the devices.

HOW HEARING LOSS CAN HURT A FAMILY

"When my mother's health was failing, the worst thing I had to deal with was her hearing loss," recalls Barbara, an only child who had to oversee her parents' complicated financial affairs in their later years. "My father had Parkinson's, and when my mother was no longer able to care for him, we had to make some tough decisions. We found a great nursing home for him, but I needed to get power of attorney and have access to their bank account. My mother didn't understand why I needed to be involved in their finances. Her eyesight wasn't good enough to read the documents from the nursing home, explaining the charges, and she couldn't hear half of what I was saying. When we tried to discuss expenses, she was outraged at the cost of everything. I think that to her, it looked like I was lying about the costs and padding the bills.

"In the end, she signed over power of attorney, but it was obvious she thought I was after their money, which just broke my heart. All I wanted was to make certain they would both have the care they needed. But I truly think she died believing I had taken their money and home for myself."

Hearing Aids Explained

If you or someone you know is in the market for a hearing aid, this chapter should help you make a smart decision. There are a number of different types of hearing aids available. The style you choose depends in part on the type of hearing loss, so the process of selecting a hearing aid begins with a visit to an otolaryngologist or ear, nose, and throat doctor (ENT). Then an audiologist can perform tests to measure various aspects of your hearing loss to determine whether hearing aids are appropriate, and if so, which type would be best.

Hearing aids can make a major difference in the lives of those with noise-induced or age-related hearing loss. If the hearing loss is due to surgery to remove a brain tumor, trauma such as a skull fracture, or meningitis, though, conventional hearing aids may not help. In such situations, a bone-anchored hearing aid (BAHA) might offer some benefit. The BAHA has received approval from the FDA for use in conductive types of hearing loss (situations where sound cannot get transmitted to the inner ear because of a malformed outer ear). This requires a minor outpatient surgical procedure, and the sound quality is actually quite good.

Concerns about cost should be discussed up front with the audiologist. Hearing aids are not inexpensive, and they are generally not covered by insurance. Typically, one hearing aid costs anywhere from $700 to $3,000; the BAHA is more expensive, with prices ranging from $10,000 to $18,000.

Because hearing aids need to be customized to an individual's needs, do not buy hearing aids through the mail or on the Internet. They may seem like bargains, but the odds are they won't do much for your hearing.

In addition, be sure to talk to your audiologist about adjustments, warranties, and the company's return policy. This last factor is especially important, because a number of companies have a "trial period" of one month when returns are accepted and refunds given. This is an outstanding feature, but don't take advantage of it too quickly. Unlike glasses, hearing aids require adjustments, sometimes repeatedly. If you have never worn a hearing aid before, you may be shocked at first by its effect on hearing. "I can hear *everything*!" is a frequent comment, for example. Many times the people who say this are not pleased. The sudden amplification of sounds that were previously not heard can be overwhelming, and it is very tempting to give up after spending hundreds—or even thousands—of dollars on an appliance that does not seem to be working. In some ways, getting a new hearing aid is like getting a new baseball mitt. The frustration of breaking in the new mitt makes you want to throw it away and go get the old one out of the garage. But give the hearing aid time to break in.

As we mentioned earlier, hearing aids are not popular to begin with. So any excuse to return them for the refund is welcome. Resist that temptation and go back to the audiologist and be brutally honest about what is not working for you. Is the size awkward? Are the on-off switches difficult to reach? Are all sounds too loud? Or are certain frequencies, such as very high or low, bothering you? Adjustments can make all the difference. It often requires several trips to the audiologist to get to the point where the hearing aids are working the way you want them to. But most patients agree that once hearing aids are fine-tuned, they are well worth the investment of money and time.

Let's take a look at some of the different types of hearing aids available today. Basically, there are four styles: the in-the-ear (ITE), behind-the-ear (BTE), in-the-canal (ITC), and completely-in-canal (CIC). In addition, there are also devices known as body aids, but these are used primarily by individuals dealing with severe hearing loss, so they are not technically hearing aids. Here's a closer look at these four:

- ITE (in-the-ear) aids are classic plastic devices that are situated in the outer ear and are completely visible. They can be equipped with extra features, like telecoils that enhance telephone sounds.
- BTE (behind-the-ear) devices are mostly tucked away behind the ear, but there is also an element called the ear-mold that sits in the outer ear and relays sound into the ear canal.
- ITC (in-the-canal) styles are tailored to each individual and are positioned inside the ear canal, where they are hard to see.

- CIC (completely-in-canal) are very tiny and fit neatly into the ear canal, making them the least obtrusive. Making adjustments with CIC or ITC models can be challenging, though, simply because of their size.

THE HEARING AID YOU THROW AWAY

Disposable hearing aids are a new item on the market. Intended for those with minimal hearing loss, these devices are offered in one size, but because they are flexible, proper fit is not a problem. Disposable hearing aids can be worn for a little more than a month and cost about forty dollars. You will still have to visit an ENT and have the audiologist perform a hearing test, but after that, a new hearing aid arrives in the mail about every forty days. Ask your audiologist or ENT about this disposable hearing device to find out if it is a viable option for you.

In addition to these classifications, there is another consideration—how the hearing aid works. For example, hearing aids are available in both analog and digital models, plus you can now choose between adjustable and programmable aids. These labels identify the electronics, or circuitry, of the hearing aid. Many people mistakenly believe that a digital hearing aid is smaller and therefore more discreet, because "digital" is a more recent, "high-tech" system. Actually, digital simply refers to a hearing aid's circuitry, or operating system, which does not make a difference in size. Digital hearing aids generally offer a wider range of adjustments than analog aids, but they are also more expensive.

So what exactly is the difference between the adjustable and programmable models? Adjustable hearing aids are built according to the information the audiologist provides the hearing aid company after you complete a hearing exam. In that sense, the adjustable hearing aids are somewhat like a pair of glasses. The eye doctor tests your vision, determines what corrections are required, and orders appropriate lenses. Similarly, the audiologist tests an individual's hearing, determines where the weaknesses lie, and takes impressions of the ear so a hearing aid can be designed to correct the problem. Unlike eyeglasses, though, the audiologist can fine-tune the hearing aid to some degree after it is built.

The settings on programmable hearing aids are established by computer, with the audiologist's input. An analog-programmable aid may offer two or more settings, to help with hearing in different situations. Digital-programmable models provide even more options.

THE POWER OF PERSISTENCE

After repeated adjustments to a digital hearing aid that simply wasn't working out, Malcolm was frustrated and ready to give up. But his fiancée convinced him to try again. "Since the digital wasn't a good experience, I decided to try an analog model," he remembers. "But the results weren't much better."

Then Malcolm began to wonder why neither one was working for him. "It just didn't make sense," he says. "Plenty of people wear hearing aids. I know people who say they changed their life. Why couldn't I find one that worked?"

Malcolm made an appointment with a different audiologist, who found that it wasn't the hearing aid—it was

Malcolm's ear canals. Both had collapsed, something that was not discovered during the initial assessment. With this knowledge, Malcolm's ENT could make new impressions, and soon he was wearing hearing aids that worked even better than he had hoped. "I see why people say they can change your life," he says. "And to think I almost gave up on hearing again."

Which hearing aid is right for you? No one but you can really answer that question, although the audiologist and/or ENT can certainly supply well-informed opinions. Joyce had been wearing hearing aids for more than a decade when she decided it was time to upgrade to a more sophisticated digital model. But after repeated adjustments, she ended up returning them. "I decided to stick with the old ones and just have the right ear put in a new case, because it never fit very well." Because of a slight bend in her ear canal which had never been noticed before, the right side of Joyce's old hearing aid always seemed awkward. The new case added a tiny extension to the microphone that extends into the ear canal, and with that little improvement, Joyce says, her hearing is as close to normal as it has been in years.

One key to success with hearing aids is allowing an appropriate amount of time to become accustomed to hearing again. People with hearing loss are so used to *not* hearing that when they try hearing aids for the first time, the initial shock of all the sounds can be overwhelming and not at all pleasant. Generally, with continued adjustments, the audiologist can modify the sounds so the hearing aids become your friend rather than a foe.

OVERCOMING THE STIGMA THAT SHOULDN'T EXIST

For years, Reuben had pretended that his hearing was just fine. Then one day the auto body shop foreman was nearly killed when a co-worker was backing a car out of the shop and Reuben didn't hear the horn honking at him. "I need a hearing aid if I'm going to keep my job," he told me. "Guys have to yell to ask me questions, I don't hear the phone ringing, and I nearly got run over. I have to do something."

The hearing aid came, Reuben seemed pleased with the results, and the next time I saw him, I asked if he was now able to hear better at the garage. "I don't know," he confessed. "I don't wear it at work, because the other guys will make fun of me."

As it turned out, Reuben first started by wearing the hearing aid at home and was impressed by how much it improved his ability to hear. But one evening when he was in a restaurant with his family, a friend came by, noticed the hearing aid, and made a thoughtless remark about how old Reuben must be if he needed help hearing. Now Reuben was afraid that his co-workers would think the same thing.

I explained to him that hearing aids are no different than glasses, which millions of people wear. Being embarrassed about hearing loss made no more sense than being ashamed about being nearsighted, I told him. The best way to overcome the stigma associated with hearing aids is to simply be up front and honest about the situation and not try to hide the fact.

It took several weeks for Reuben to face his co-workers with the hearing aid in place, but afterward he was glad he did. "I could not believe what a difference it made at work," he told me. "It's always so noisy in the garage, that's probably why my hearing is so bad to begin with.

But now I can understand the questions the guys are asking, I hear the phone ringing, and I don't have to worry about getting run over."

But what about his co-workers' attitude? I asked. Did anyone make fun of him or tell him he must be getting old? Reuben was happy to explain that he decided to head them off. The first day he wore the hearing aid, he announced it to everyone, telling them he would now be able to hear them if they talked about him or gave him a hard time behind his back. "And that did it," he said proudly. "They congratulated me on doing something about it, and we all went back to work."

A Look at Cochlear Implants

A cochlear implant is designed to provide auditory information to severely and profoundly hearing-impaired individuals whose ability to understand speech with a hearing aid is severely restricted. In general, a candidate for cochlear implants must have a severe to profound hearing loss, and receive little to no benefit from a hearing aid. A surgeon assesses whether or not an individual is an appropriate candidate. Because learning to live with a cochlear implant can be challenging, a patient needs to be highly motivated, have a strong support system consisting of family and friends, and have reasonable expectations as well.

The cochlear implant consists of a device that is placed beneath the skin behind the ear (into the mastoid cavity) during the surgical procedure. An electrode array is part of this internal component, and it is placed into the cochlea. Some people can feel the device behind the ear, and it may become more noticeable over time, particularly as the post-surgery swelling decreases.

The cochlear implant also requires the individual to wear an external processor that can be worn in a pocket, on the waistband, or on a belt, as well as behind the ear. The processor includes several components, among them a microphone, which receives the acoustic signal and sends it to the processor.

When a cochlear implant is in place, the recipient should be able to hear as soon as the processor is activated, but it can take time for the person to understand speech through the implant, especially if the individual has not been able to hear for some time. The auditory signal will not sound the same way that is remembered, and music may not sound the same, either. Learning to hear again with a cochlear implant takes some time, and each individual must practice listening with the device on a regular basis. But people who have reasonable expectations and are patient with the learning process say that the devices have changed their lives.

FIFTEEN QUESTIONS TO ASK THE ENT OR AUDIOLOGIST ABOUT HEARING AIDS

1. What kind of hearing loss do I have?
2. Can hearing aids help correct my hearing loss?
3. Which hearing aids are best for this kind of hearing loss?
4. What special features do these hearing aids offer?
5. Are there downsides involved with these aids, and if so, what are they?
6. How long do these kinds of hearing aids usually last?
7. How much should I expect to pay for these hearing aids?
8. How long have these hearing aids been on the market, and are they popular with your other patients?

9. Are they covered by a warranty, and if so, how long does it last, and can it be extended?
10. Do these aids require special care?
11. Are they returnable? How long do I have to decide that they are not for me?
12. What can I expect when I first try these hearing aids?
13. How many adjustments does it typically take to get these hearing aids in proper working order?
14. Where are the adjustments made, and does the company provide "loaners" if these need to be repaired?
15. How long should I wait before determining that these hearing aids are not for me?

High-Tech Ears: Assistive Listening Technology

Hearing aids and cochlear implants are not the only options when it comes to helping those with hearing loss. A wide range of products known as assistive listening devices (ALDs) can be used with or without hearing aids to amplify sounds or to improve hearing when circumstances are less than ideal.

The personal FM system, for example, relays sounds to a headset or hearing aid, and can be helpful in public places or situations where the acoustics make hearing difficult, such as restaurants, conference rooms, museums, and theaters. Telephone amplifying devices and amplified answering machines, alarm clocks, smoke detectors, and computers can also ease difficulties faced by those with hearing loss. In addition, infrared systems designed for in-home use make it possible to keep the television volume at a level that is comfortable for everyone, while the individual with a hearing problem wears a receiver with adjustable volume.

For anyone with hearing loss, ALDs can restore a great deal of normalcy to everyday living. Ask your ENT or audiologist for recommendations.

((**14**))

CLOSING REMARKS

Not so long ago, devices like cochlear implants and partially implantable hearing aids, such as the BAHA, only existed as concepts. Today, these devices are enabling individuals with serious hearing loss to live normal lives again. In the future, improvement in speech recognition will make the process of adjusting to these devices far easier.

Meanwhile, hearing loss remedies on the horizon promise to revolutionize the treatment of both hearing loss and deafness. Already, researchers are implanting new hair cells in the cochlea and encouraging existing hair cells to regenerate, a process never before achieved in mammals. Right now the work is experimental, but the foundation is being created for advances in hearing technology that no one could have imagined just a few years ago.

Regardless of the technological advances that may occur in the future, right now it makes sense to protect your hearing. When it comes to fighting hearing loss, the knowledge presented in this book is the ultimate weapon. By reading this book, you have become familiar with the amazing, intricate process of hearing. As you have seen, the auditory system is made up of resilient but fragile components, such as the hair cells, which need to be shielded from loud noises and nurtured with appropriate substances to remain in top working order.

The Save Your Hearing Now Program is designed to do just that. Based on cutting-edge research, the four steps provide a flexible, easy-to-follow framework. Scientifically proven antioxidant supplements and nutrients to enhance mitochondrial function are the program's foundation. A Mediterranean-style meal plan, based on research showing the benefits of a diet rich in fruits, vegetables, whole grains, lean proteins, and good fats, enhances the supplements' work by providing additional nutrients. Physical activity, meanwhile, stimulates circulation, which relays nutrients throughout the auditory system, as well as the rest of the body. Furthermore, these three steps can also slow the aging process, an essential element in protecting against hearing loss and restoring damaged hair cells to good health.

Finally, by using devices that protect the ears during exposure to noise and seeking out some quiet time each day, you can reduce damage to the auditory system and make the first three Save Your Hearing Now elements even more effective. In addition, cutting back on noise exposure also decreases stress and other negative health effects linked to noise pollution.

While the Save Your Hearing Now Program is designed to be user-friendly, I encourage you to consult with a physician or ENT to discuss your special hearing difficulties and enlist his or her assistance in further preventing hearing loss.

Remember that the healing process requires time, so keep expectations reasonable and focus on staying with the program. The key to success, as I have had to remind more than a few patients, is in the synergy created when all four elements are combined. Tricia is an excellent example. Only in her early forties, Tricia had been working as a concert promoter in the music industry for two decades. The repeated exposure to hours of rehearsals followed by high-volume performances by rock bands had robbed Tricia of a great deal of her hearing. In fact, it was surprising she was not in much worse shape, considering the punishment her ears had endured. Since she was still fairly young and healthy—plus no longer in the music industry—I felt the program could work for her. But she was less than thrilled at my suggestions to make lifestyle changes. Years of eating on the road had left Tricia with a serious fast-food addiction. And her schedule had been erratic for so long that she hadn't really exercised since high school physical education classes.

"I'm forty-four, my kids are eleven and nine, and I'm a single mother," she explained, "working as a Realtor, on the go all day. I don't know how to find time to exercise and cook—no way!"

We talked about the fact that if she didn't do something about her hearing loss soon, Tricia would very likely be wearing hearing aids in the near future. At that point, she started to pay attention. "My dad has a hearing aid, and he's not happy about it," she explained. "You're right. Maybe I should do something before it's too late."

Adding supplements to her day was not a problem, but Tricia was determined to avoid a hearing aid for as long as possible, so she set aside time every morning to go for a walk. That way, she said, her physical activity was out of the way and she could concentrate on work the rest of the day. Then she enlisted her children's help with meal planning, because she realized they would benefit from a better diet, too. Everyone picked out favorite fruits and vegetables at the market, and they made a deal to try one new type of produce every week. With the refrigerator well stocked, and different types of whole grains in the cupboard, Tricia invested in a slow cooker that made it easy to have hot soups, stews, and rice dishes at the end of the day. Finally, Tricia decided to devote her driving time to silence. "The news is usually pretty upsetting anyway, so now I turn off the radio and just let my ears—and emotions—rest."

After a few months on the program, Tricia reported that things were improving all around. Her children were enjoying their home-cooked meals and were even willing to help out with planning and preparation. The daily walks and quiet time in the car were working, too, because both gave Tricia time to clear her mind and plan ahead. And the supplements were doing their job. Although she had been using a telephone with adjustable voice control to help her hear better, Tricia had still been having difficulty with phone conversations before starting on the program. "But now I don't have to ask clients to repeat themselves constantly on the phone," she explained. "It really makes my life easier and a lot less stressful."

New research is continually revealing the healing power of nutrients, and increasingly, medical experts are using these natural substances to treat common disorders that conventional medicine cannot remedy. As more patients and doctors alike discover the effectiveness of alternative therapies, the way we approach and treat a wide range of health conditions, including hearing loss, is changing. I am certain that many people can preserve their hearing, and possibly even improve it, by following the Save Your Hearing Now Program. And I hope that you are among them.

RESOURCES

These are just a few of the many organizations and Web sites devoted to various aspects of hearing and/or health.

IN THE UNITED STATES

Alexander Graham Bell Association for the Deaf and Hard of Hearing (AG Bell)
3417 Volta Place, NW
Washington, DC 20007-2778
Voice: 202-337-5220
Toll-free voice: 866-337-5220
TTY: 202-337-5221
Fax: 202-337-8314
Web site: www.agbell.org
E-mail: info@agbell.org

American Academy of Audiology (AAA)
11730 Plaza America Drive, Suite 300
Reston, VA 20190
Voice: 703-790-8466
Toll-free voice: 800-222-2336
TTY: 703-790-8466
Fax: 703-790-8631
Web site: www.audiology.org
E-mail: info@audiology.org

**American Academy of Otolaryngology–Head and
Neck Surgery (AAO-HNS)**
One Prince Street
Alexandria, VA 22314-3357
Voice: 703-836-4444
TTY: 703-519-1585
Fax: 703-683-5100
Web site: www.entnet.org
E-mail: webmaster@entnet.org

**American Association of Retired Persons (AARP)
Disability Initiative**
601 E Street, NW
Washington, DC 20049
Toll-free: 800-424-3410
Toll-free TTY: 877-434-7598
Fax: 202-434-6406
Web site: www.aarp.org
E-mail: member@aarp.org

American Speech-Language–Hearing Association (ASHA)
10801 Rockville Pike
Rockville, MD 20852
Voice: 301-897-5700
Toll-free voice: 800-638-8255
TTY: 301-897-0157

Fax: 301-571-0457
Web site: www.asha.org
E-mail: actioncenter@asha.org

American Tinnitus Association
P.O. Box 5
Portland, OR 97207-0005
Voice: 503-248-9985
Toll-free voice: 800-634-8978
Fax: 503-248-0024
Web site: www.ata.org
E-mail: tinnitus@ata.org

Better Hearing Institute (BHI)
515 King Street, Suite 420
Alexandria, VA 22314
Voice: 703-684-3391
Toll-free voice: 800-EAR-WELL (800-327-9355)
Fax: 703-684-6048
Web site: www.betterhearing.org
E-mail: mail@betterhearing.org

HEAR NOW
6700 Washington Avenue S
Eden Prairie, MN 55344
Toll-free voice: 800-648-4327
Fax: 952-828-6946
Web site: www.sotheworldmayhear.org
E-mail: joanita@sotheworldmayhear.org

Hearing Industries Association (HIA)
515 King Street, Suite 420
Alexandria, VA 22314
Voice: 703-684-5744
Fax: 703-684-6048
Web site: www.hearing.org
E-mail: crogin@clarionmanagement.com

**National Institute on Deafness and Other
Communication Disorders**
National Institutes of Health
31 Center Drive, MSC 2320
Bethesda, MD 20892-2320
Web site: http://www.nidcd.nih.gov
E-mail: nidcdinfo@nidcd.nih.gov

This organization sponsors Wise Ears®, a national campaign to reduce noise-induced hearing loss. Learn more at http://www.nidcd.nih.gov/health/wise/index.asp.

Occupational Safety and Health Administration (OSHA)
Oversees workplace safety, including noise levels.
http://www.osha.gov

Self Help for the Hard of Hearing (SHHH)
7910 Woodmont Avenue, Suite 1200
Bethesda, MD 20814
Voice: 301-657-2238
TTY: 301-657-2249
Fax: 301-913-9413
Web site: http://www.shhh.org

INTERNATIONAL

Deaf Cultures and Sign Languages of the World
A huge list of international agencies and organizations including Internet addresses in more than 145 countries.
www.theinterpretersfriend.com/indj/dcoew.html#world

Hearing International
In cooperation with the World Health Organization (WHO) and other agencies, this nongovernmental organization focuses on various hearing-loss-related topics, such as ear infections, noise-induced hearing loss, drug-induced hearing loss, and hereditary deafness.
www.med.teikyo-u.ac.jp/~hi-japan/HomePage.html

International Federation of Hard of Hearing People (IFHOHP)

In conjunction with the International Federation for Hard of Hearing Young People, the IFHOHP encourages information exchange between all organizations devoted to issues for the hard of hearing.

www.ifhoh.org

International Federation of Oto-Rhino-Laryngological Societies (IFOS)

Working with the World Health Organization (WHO), this group focuses on otorhinolaryngological issues and needs, as well as methods of treating and dealing with them.

www.ifosworld.org

International Society of Audiology (ISA)

An organization for people in the audiology profession, ISA functions as a clearinghouse for information and education, with a separate branch managing philanthropic ventures.

www.isa-audiology.org

World Health Organization Prevention of Deafness and Hearing Impairment

Under the auspices of the United Nations, this agency works with member states on reducing hearing loss and deafness all over the world.

www.who.int/noncommunicable_diseases/about/pbd/en
www.wfdeaf.org

HIGH-FREQUENCY DOG TRAINING DEVICES

Pet Agree

http://www.boxess.com/zap.htm

Dressler Dog Training
http://www.dresslersdog.com/Barktrain.html

EXERCISE

American College of Sports Medicine
Downloadable (PDF format) brochures on exercise and some nutrition information, as well as searchable database for personal training specialists.
http://www.acsm.org

NUTRITION AND ITS LINK TO HEALTH

American Dietetic Association
www.eatright.org/Public

SUPPLEMENT SUPPLIERS

Anti-Aging/Energy Formula by Body Language Vitamin Company
Part of a comprehensive line of nutritional supplements created by Dr. Michael D. Seidman to protect and enhance hearing, as well as improve overall health. The Anti-Aging/Energy Formula contains ALA, ALC, Coenzyme Q10, and glutathione. Available online at
www.bodylanguagevitamin.com.

Acety-l-Carnitine and Alpha Lipoic Acid from Source Naturals
A combination of these two antioxidants from a well-known nutritional supplement manufacturer with a wide range of products. Available in health food stores nationwide and at various online retailers.
www.sourcenaturals.com.

Anti-Aging & Energy Complex from ViSalus Science

Designed by Dr. Michael D. Seidman, this combination of ALA, ALC, Coenzyme Q10, and glutathione was created to fight aging at the cellular level. This combination of antioxidants is also recommended for preserving and protecting hearing. Available at www.visalus.com, with other complementary products.

Tinnitus Formulas from Arches

Available in different formulations (Relief, Stress, and B_{12}), these supplements have been shown to be highly effective in reducing tinnitus in thousands of individuals. They are recommended by more than a thousand otolaryngologists and endorsed by Dr. Seidman.

www.tinnitusformula.com.

RESOURCES FOR COCHLEAR IMPLANTS

Cochlear Americas

400 Inverness Parkway, Ste. 400
Englewood, CO 80112
(800) 790-9010
Telephone: 303-792-9025
Fax: 303-792-9025
www.cochlear.com

MED-EL Corporation (North America)

2222 East Highway 54,
Beta Building Suite 180
Durham, NC 27713
Telephone: 919-572-2222
Fax: 919-484-9229
Toll Free: (888) MED-EL-CI (633-3524)
www.medel.com
E-mail: implants@medelus.com

Advanced Bionics Corporation
12740 San Fernando Road
Sylmar, CA 91342
Telephone: 661-362-1400
Toll Free: 800-678-2575
TTY: 800-678-3575
Fax: 661-362-1500
www.cochlearimplant.com
E-mail: info@advancedbionics.com

REFERENCES

Chapter Three: How Aging Affects Hearing and What We Can Do About It

1. Wallace DC, "Mitochondrial genetics: A paradigm for ageing and degenerative diseases?" *Science* 1992; 256:628–32.

2. Granville DJ, Gottlieb RA, "Mitochondria: Regulators of cell death and survival," *Scientific World Journal* 2002; Vol. 2: 1569–78.

3. Johnsson LG, Hawkins JE Jr., "Vascular changes in the human inner ear associated with aging," *Annals of Otology, Rhinology & Laryngology* 1972 Jun; 81 (3): 361–76.

4. Seidman MD, Khan MJ, Dolan D, et al., "Age related differences in cochlear microcirculation and auditory brain stem responses," presented at the 19th Midwinter Research Meeting of the Association for Research in Otolaryngology, 1996, St. Petersburg, FL. Miller JM, Marks NJ, Goodwin PC, "Laser Doppler measurements of cochlear blood flow," *Hearing Research* 1983 Sep; 11 (3): 385–94.

5. Semsei I, Rao G, Richardson A, "Changes in the expression of superoxide dismutase and catalase as a function of age and dietary restriction," *Biochemical and Biophysical Research Communication* 1989 Oct 31; 164 (2): 620–25.

6. Bai U, Seidman MD, Hinojosa R, Quirk WS, "Mitochondrial DNA deletions associated with aging and possibly presbycusis: A human archival temporal bone study," *American Journal of Otology* 1997 Jul; 18 (4): 449–53.

7. Seidman MD, Bai U, Khan MJ, Quirk WS, "Mitochondrial DNA deletions associated with aging and presbyacusis," *Archives of Otolaryngology* 1997 Oct; 123:1039–45.

8. Seidman MD, "Effects of dietary restriction and antioxidants on presbyacusis," *Laryngoscope* 2000 May; 110 (5 pt 1): 727–38.

9. Seidman MD, Khan MJ, Bai U, Shirwany N, Quirk WS, "Biologic activity of mitochondrial metabolites on aging and age-related hearing loss," *American Journal of Otology* 2000 Mar; 21(2): 161–67.

10. Kujala UM, Kaprio J, Koskenvuo M, "Modifiable risk factors as predictors of all-cause mortality: The roles of genetics and childhood environment," *American Journal of Epidemiology* 2002 Dec 1; 156 (11): 985–93.

11. Lee CK, Weindruch R, Prolla TA, "Gene-expression profile of the ageing brain in mice," *Nature Genetics* 2000 Jul; 25 (3): 294–97.

12. Fraser GE, Singh PN, Bennett H, "Variables associated with cognitive function in elderly California Seventh-Day Adventists," *American Journal of Epidemiology* 1996 Jun 15; 143 (12): 1181–90. Kidd PM, "Parkinson's disease as multifactorial oxidative neurodegeneration: implications for integrative management," *Alternative Medicine Review* 2000 Dec; 5 (6): 502–29.

13. Fang J, Wylie-Rosett J, Alderman MH, "Exercise and cardiovascular outcomes by hypertensive status: NHANES I epidemiological follow-up study, 1971–1992," *American Journal of Hypertension* 2005 Jun; 18 (6): 751–78.

14. Torre P 3rd, Cruickshanks KJ, Klein BE, Klein R, Nondahl DM, "The association between cardiovascular disease and cochlear function in older adults," *Journal of Speech, Language and Hearing Research* 2005 Apr; 48 (2): 473–81.

Chapter Four: Noise and Other Hearing Damage Culprits

1. Ganesalingam R, Radomskij P, Lo S, Knight JF, Prasher D, "Noise on London Underground Trains and Its Effect on Passengers' Cochlear Function," presented at the British Academy of Audiology 2004 Conference.

2. Stansfeld S, Haines M, Brown B, "Noise and health in the urban environment," *Review of Environmental Health* 2000 Jan–Jun; 15 (1–2): 43–82. Matsui T, Matsuno T, Ashimine K, Miyakita T, Hiramatsu K, Yamamoto T, "Association between the rates of low birthweight and/or preterm infants and aircraft noise exposure," *Nippon Eiseigaku Zasshi* 2003 Sep; 58 (3): 385–94.

3. Bremmer P, Byers JF, Kiehl E, "Noise and the premature infant: Physiological effects and practice implications," *Journal of Obstetric, Gynecologic and Neonatal Nursing* 2003 Jul–Aug; 32 (4): 447–54.

4. Niskar, AS, Kieszak SM, Holmes AE, Esteban F, Rubin C, Brody DJ, "Estimated prevalence of noise-induced hearing threshold shifts among children 6 to 19 years of age: The Third National Health and Nutrition Examination Survey, 1988–1994, United States," *Pediatrics* 2001 Jul; 108 (1): 40–43.

5. Housing Survey information from *Noise Effects Handbook: A Desk Reference to Health and Welfare Effects of Noise*, Office of the Scientific Assistant, Office of Noise Abatement and Control, U.S. Environmental Protection Agency, Oct 1979, rev. Jul 1981.

6. Von Eiff AW, Friedrich G, Langewitz W, Neus H, Ruddel H, Schirmer G, Schulte W, "Traffic noise and hypertension risk: Hypothalamus theory of essential hypertension: Second communication (author's transl)," *MMW Munchener Medizinische Wochenschrift* 1981 Mar 13; 123 (11): 420–24.

7. German studies presented at the 2004 European Society of Cardiology Congress.

8. Holand S, Girard A, Meyer-Bisch C, Eighozi JL, "Cardiovascular responses to acoustic startle stimulus in man," *Archives des Maladies du Coeur et Vaisseaux* 1999 Aug; 92 (8): 1127–31.

9. Hygge S, Evans GW, Bullinger M, "A prospective study of some effects of aircraft noise on cognitive performance in schoolchildren," *Psychological Science* 2002 Sep; 13 (5): 469–74.

10. Evans GW, Lercher P, Meis M, Ising H, Kofler WW, "Community noise exposure and stress in children," *Journal of the Acoustical Society of America* 2001 Mar; 109 (3): 1023–27.

11. Persson Waye K, Bengtsson J, Kjellberg A, Benton S, "Low frequency noise 'pollution' interferes with performance," *Noise Health* 2001; 4 (13): 33–49.

CHAPTER SIX: STEP ONE: THE NUTRIENTS YOU NEED

1. "Medical spending continues to rise at a strong pace," *Wall Street Journal* 2005 Jun 21; A2.

2. Zandi PP, Anthony JC, Khachaturian AS, et al., "Reduced risk of Alzheimer disease in users of antioxidant vitamin supplements: The Cache County Study," *Archives of Neurology* 2004 Jan; 61 (1): 82–88.

3. Church TS, Earnest CP, Wood KA, et al., "Reduction of C-reactive protein levels through use of a multivitamin," *American Journal of Medicine* 2003 Dec 15; 115 (9): 702–77.

4. Bendich A, "Micronutrients in women's health and immune function," *Nutrition* 2001 Oct; 17 (10): 858–67.

5. McKenzie J, "Health report," *World News Tonight with Peter Jennings*, Sep 29, 1997.

6. Schonheit K, Gille L, Nohl H, "Effect of alpha-lipoic acid and dihydrolipoic acid on ischemia/reperfusion injury of the heart and heart mitochondria," *Biochimica and Biophysica Acta* 1995 Jun 9; 1271 (2–3): 335–42.

7. Ziegler D, Reljanovic M, Mehnert H, Gries FA, "Alpha-lipoic acid in the treatment of diabetic polyneuropathy in Germany: Current evidence from clinical trials," *Experimental and Clinical Endocrinology and Diabetes* 1999; 107 (7): 421–30.

8. Konrad T, Vicini P, Kusterer K, Hoflich A, et al., "Alpha-lipoic acid treatment decreases serum lactate and pyruvate concentrations and improves glucose effectiveness in lean and obese patients with type 2 diabetes," *Diabetes Care* 1999 Feb; 22 (2): 280–87.

9. Bustamante J, Lodge JK, Marcocci L, Tritschler HJ, et al., "Alpha-lipoic acid in liver metabolism and disease," *Free Radical Biology and Medicine* 1998 Apr; 24 (6): 1023–39.

10. Patrick L, "Nutrients and HIV: Part three—N-acetylcysteine; alpha-lipoic acid, L-glutamine, and L-carnitine," *Alternative Medicine Review* 2000 Aug; 5 (4): 290–305.

11. "Monograph: Alpha-lipoic acid," *Alternative Medicine Review* 1998 Aug; 3 (4): 308–11.

12. Markowska AL, Ingram DK, Barnes CA, Spangler EL, et al., "Acetyl-L-carnitine: Effects on mortality, pathology and sensory-motor performance in aging rats," *Neurobiology of Aging* 1990 Sep–Oct; 11 (5): 491–98. Paradies G, Ruggiero FM, Petrosillo G, Gadaleta MN, et al., "Carnitine-acetylcarnitine translocase activity in cardiac mitochondria from aged rats: The effect of acetyl-L-carnitine," *Mechanics of Ageing and Development* 1995 Oct 13; 84 (2): 103–12. Ando S, Tadenuma T, Tanaka Y, Fukui F, et al., "Enhancement of learning capacity and cholinergic synaptic function by carnitine in aging rats," *Journal of Neuroscience Research* 2001 Oct 15; 66 (2): 266–71. Pettegrew JW, Levine J, McClure RJ, "Acetyl-L-carnitine physical-chemical, metabolic, and therapeutic properties: Relevance for its mode of action in Alzheimer's disease and geriatric depression," *Molecular Psychiatry* 2000 Nov; 5 (6): 616–32. "Acetyl-L-carnitine," *Alternative Medicine Review* 1999 Dec; 4 (6): 438–41.

13. Kopke R, Bielefeld E, Liu J, Zheng J, Jackson R, Henderson D, Coleman JK, "Prevention of impulse noise-induced hearing loss with antioxidants," *Acta Oto-laryngologica* 2005 Mar; 125 (3): 235–43.

14. Liu J, Head E, Gharib AM, Yuan W, et al., "Memory loss in old rats is associated with brain mitochondrial decay and RNA/DNA oxidation: Partial reversal by feeding acetyl-L-carnitine and/or R-alpha-lipoic acid," *Proceedings of the National Academy of Sciences USA* 2002 May 14; 99 (10): 7184–85. Hagen TM, Liu J, Lykkesfeldt J, Wehr CM, et al., "Feeding acetyl-L-carnitine and lipoic acid to old rats significantly improves metabolic function while decreasing oxidative stress," *Proceedings of the National Academy of Sciences USA* 2002 Feb 19; 99 (4): 1870–75. Hagen TM, Moreau R, Suh JH, Visioli F, "Mitochondrial decay in the aging rat heart: Evidence for improvement by dietary supplementation with acetyl-L-carnitine and/or lipoic acid," *Annals of the New York Academy of Science* 2002 Apr; 959: 491–507.

15. Angeli SI, Liu XZ, Yan D, Balkany T, Telischi F, "Coenzyme Q10 treatment of patients with a 7445A→G mitochondrial DNA mutation stops the progression of hearing loss," *Acta Oto-laryngologica* 2005 May; 125 (5): 510–12.

16. Ohinata Y, Yamasoba T, Schacht J, Miller JM, "Glutathione limits noise-induced hearing loss," *Hearing Research* 2000 Aug; 146 (1–2): 28–34. Campbell KC, Larsen DL, Meech RP, Rybak LP, Hughes LF, "Glutathione ester but not glutathione protects against cisplatin-induced ototoxicity in a rat model," *Journal of the American Academy of Audiology* 2003 April; 14 (3): 124–33.

17. Houston DK, Johnson MA, Nozza RJ, Gunter EW, Shea KJ, Cutler GM, Edmonds JT, "Age-related hearing loss, vitamin B_{12}, and folate in elderly women," *American Journal of Clinical Nutrition* 1999 Mar; 69 (3): 564–71.

18. Sharabi A, Cohen E, Sulkes J, Garty M, "Replacement therapy for vitamin B_{12} deficiency: Comparison between the sublingual and oral route," *British Journal of Clinical Pharmacology* 2003 Dec; 56 (6): 635–38.

19. Seidman MD, Khan MJ, Tang WX, Quirk WS, "Influence of lecithin on mitochondrial DNA and age-related hearing loss," *Otolaryngology, Head and Neck Surgery* 2002 Sep; 127 (3): 138–44.

20. Duan M, Qiu J, Laurell G, Olofsson A, Counter SA, Borg E, "Dose and time-dependent protection of the antioxidant N-L-acetylcysteine against impulse noise trauma," *Hearing Research* 2004 Jun; 192 (1–2): 1–9. Kopke R, Bielefeld E, Liu J, Zheng J, Jackson R, Henderson D, Coleman JK, "Prevention of impulse noise-induced hearing loss with antioxidants," *Acta Oto-laryngologica* 2005 Mar; 125 (3): 235–43.

21. Seidman M, Babu S, Tang W, Naem E, Quirk WS, "Effects of resveratrol on acoustic trauma," *Otolaryngology, Head and Neck Surgery* 2003 Nov; 129 (5): 463–70.

22. Nihei T, Miura Y, Yagasaki K, "Inhibitory effect of resveratrol on proteinuria, hypoalbuminemia and hyperlipidemia in nephritic rats," *Life Sciences* 2001 May 11; 68 (25): 2845–52.

23. Lefebvre P, Malgrange B, Van de Water T, Moonen G, "Jean Marquet Award: Regeneration of the neurosensory structures in the mammalian inner ear," *Acta Oto-Rhino-Laryngologica Belgica* 1997; 51 (1): 1–10.

24. McFadden SL, Woo JM, Michalak N, Ding D, "Dietary vitamin C supplementation reduces noise-induced hearing loss in guinea pigs," *Hearing Research* 2005 Apr; 202 (1–2): 200–08.

25. Brookes GB, "Vitamin D deficiency—a new cause of cochlear deafness," *Journal of Laryngology and Otology* 1983 May; 97 (5): 405–20. Brookes GB, "Vitamin D deficiency and deafness: 1984 update," *American Journal of Otology* 1985 Jan; 6 (1): 102–7. Brookes GB, "Vitamin D deficiency and otosclerosis," *Otolaryngology, Head and Neck Surgery* 1985 Jun; 93 (3): 313–21.

26. Miller ER 3rd, Pastor-Barriuso R, Dalal D, Riemersma RA, Appel LJ, Guallar E, "Meta-analysis: High-dosage vitamin E supplementation may increase all-cause mortality," *Annals of Internal Medicine* 2005 Jan 4; 142 (1): 37–46.

27. Attias J, Sapir S, Bresloff I, et al., "Reduction in noise-induced temporary threshold shift in humans following oral magnesium intake," *Clinics in Otolaryngology and Allied Sciences* 2004 Dec; 29 (6): 635–41.

CHAPTER SEVEN: STEP TWO: A SOUND DIET STRATEGY

1. Thorpe KE, Florence CS, Howard DH, Joski P, "The impact of obesity on rising medical spending," *Health Affairs* 2004 Jul–Dec; Suppl Web Exclusives: W4-480-6.

2. Patterson RE, Frank LL, Kristal AR, White E, "A comprehensive examination of health conditions associated with obesity in older adults," *American Journal of Preventive Medicine* 2004 Dec; 27 (5): 385–90.

3. Gustafson D, Lissner L, Bengtsson C, et al., "A 24-year follow-up of body mass index and cerebral atrophy," *Neurology* 2004 Nov 23; 63 (10): 1876–81.

4. Valdes AM, Andrew T, Gardner JP, Kimura M, Oelsner E, Cherkas IF, Aviv A, Spector TD, "Obesity, cigarette smoking, and telomere length in women," *Lancet* 2005 Aug 20–26; 366 (9486): 662–4.

5. Trichopoulou A, Costacou T, Bamia C, Trichopoulos D, "Adherence to a Mediterranean diet and survival in a Greek population," *New England Journal of Medicine* 2003 Jun 26; 348 (26): 2599–608.

6. Curl CL, Fenske RA, Elgethun K, "Organophosphorus pesticide exposure of urban and suburban preschool children with organic and conventional diets," *Environmental Health Perspectives* 2003 Mar; 111 (3): 377–82.

7. Hashimoto F, Ono M, Masuoka C, Ito Y, et al., "Evaluation of the anti-oxidative effect (in vitro) of tea polyphenols," *Bioscience, Biotechnology and Biochemistry* 2003 Feb; 67 (2): 396–401.

8. Dulloo AG, Duret C, Rohrer D, Girardier L, et al., "Efficacy of a green tea extract rich in catechin polyphenols and caffeine in increasing 24-h energy expenditure and fat oxidation in humans," *American Journal of Clinical Nutrition* 1999 Dec; 70 (6): 1040–45.

9. Rumpler W, Seale J, Clevidence B, Judd J, et al., "Oolong tea increases metabolic rate and fat oxidation in men," *Journal of Nutrition* 2001 Nov; 131 (11): 2848–52.

10. Burton-Freeman B, Davis PA, Schneeman BO, "Plasma chole-cystokinin is associated with subjective measures of satiety in women," *American Journal of Clinical Nutrition* 2002 Sep; 76 (3): 659–67.

11. Davy BM, Davy KP, Ho RC, Beske SD, et al., "High-fiber oat cereal compared with wheat cereal consumption favorably alters LDL-cholesterol subclass and particle numbers in middle-aged and older men," *American Journal of Clinical Nutrition* 2002 Aug; 76 (2): 351–58.

12. Griel AE, Eissenstat B, Juturu V, Hsieh G, Kris-Etherton PM, "Improved diet quality with peanut consumption," *Journal of the American College of Nutrition* 2004 Dec; 23 (6): 660–68.

13. DeLorgeril M, Salen P, Martin JL, Monjaud I, Delaye J, Mamelle N, "Mediterranean diet, traditional risk factors, and the rate of cardiovascular complications after myocardial infarction: Final report of the Lyon Diet Heart Study," *Circulation* 1999 Feb 16; 99 (6): 779–85.

14. Morris MC, Manson JE, Rosner B, Buring JE, Willett WC, Hennekens CH, "Fish consumption and cardiovascular disease in the Physicians' Health Study: A prospective study," *American Journal of Epidemiology* 1995 Jul 15; 142 (2): 166–75.

15. Hu FB, Bronner L, Willett WC, Stampfer MJ, et al., "Fish and omega 3 fatty acid intake and risk of coronary heart disease in women," *Journal of the American Medical Association* 2002 Apr 10; 287 (14): 1815–21.

16. Hites RA, Foran JA, Carpenter DO, et al., "Global Assessment of Organic Contaminants in Farmed Salmon," *Science* 2004 Jan 303; (5655): 226–229.

17. Morrill AC, Chinn CD, "The obesity epidemic in the United States," *Journal of Public Health Policy* 2004; 25 (3–4): 353–66.

18. University of Texas Health Science Center at San Antonio study of diet soda and weight presented June 12, 2005, at the American Diabetes Association's 65th Annual Scientific Sessions, San Diego, CA.

19. Rolls BJ, Morris EL, Roe LS, "Portion size of food affects energy intake in normal-weight and overweight men and women," *American Journal of Clinical Nutrition* 2002 Dec; 76 (6): 1207–13.

20. Wardle J, Guthrie C, Sanderson S, et al., "Food and activity preferences in children of lean and obese parents," *International Journal of Obesity and Related Metabolic Disorders* 2001 Jul; 25 (7): 971–77.

21. Bell EA, Rolls BJ, "Energy density of foods affects energy intake across multiple levels of fat content in lean and obese women," *American Journal of Clinical Nutrition* 2001 Jun; 73 (6): 1010–18.

22. Rolls BJ, Roe LS, Meengs JS, "Salad and satiety: Energy density and portion size of a first-course salad affect energy intake at lunch," *Journal of the American Dietetic Association* 2004 Oct; 104 (10): 1570–76.

23. Knoops KT, de Groot LC, Kromhout D, Perrin AE, Moreiras-Varela O, Menotti A, van Staveren WA, "Mediterranean diet, lifestyle factors, and 10-year mortality in elderly European men and women: The HALE project," *Journal of the American Medical Association* 2004 Sep 22; 292 (12): 1433–39.

24. Layman DK, "Protein quantity and quality at levels above the RDA improves adult weight loss," *Journal of the American College of Nutrition* 2004 Dec; 23 (6 Suppl): 631S–636S.

25. Serra-Majem L, de la Cruz JN, Ribas L, Salleras L, "Mediterranean diet and health: Is all the secret in olive oil?" *Pathophysiology, Haemostat and Thrombosis* 2003 Sep–2004 Dec; 33 (5–6): 461–65.

CHAPTER EIGHT: STEP THREE: MOVE IT!

1.Wilsont WJ, Herbstein N, "The role of music intensity in aerobics: Implications for hearing conservation," *Journal of the American Academy of Audiology* 2003; 14 (1): 29–38.

2. Tudor-Locke C, Bassett DR, "How many steps/day are enough? Preliminary pedometer indices for public health," *Sports Medicine* 2004; 34 (1): 1–8.

3. Pedometer study presented at the American College of Sports Medicine annual meeting, Jun 2004, Indianapolis, IN.

4. Tsang WW, Hui-Chan CW, "Effect of 4- and 8-wk intensive tai chi training on balance control in the elderly," *Medicine & Science in Sports & Exercise* 2004 Apr; 36 (4): 648–57.

CHAPTER NINE: STEP FOUR: ALL ABOUT EAR PROTECTION

1. Lopez HH, Bracha AS, Bracha HS, "Evidence based complementary intervention for insomnia," *Hawaii Medical Journal* 2002 Sep; 61 (9): 192, 213.

CHAPTER ELEVEN: SO LONG, STRESS, AND GOOD-BYE, BLUES!

1. Epel ES, Blackburn EH, Lin J, et al., "Accelerated telomere shortening in response to life stress," *Proceedings of the National Academy of Sciences USA* 2004 Dec 7; 101 (49): 17312–15; e-pub 2004 Dec 1.

2. Bradbury J, Myers SP, Oliver C, "An adaptogenic role for omega-3 fatty acids in stress: A randomized placebo controlled double-blind intervention study (pilot)," *Nutrition Journal* 2004 Nov 28; 3 (1): 20.

3. Smith JC, Joyce CA, "Mozart versus New Age music: Relaxation states, stress, and ABC relaxation theory," *Journal of Music Therapy* 2004 Fall; 41 (3): 215–24.

4. Twins stress study presented at the 53rd Scientific Session of the American College of Cardiology, Mar 8, 2004, New Orleans, LA.

5. Warden SJ, Robling AG, Sanders MS, et al., "Inhibition of the serotonin transporter (5-HTT) reduces bone accrual during growth," *Endocrinology* 2004 Nov 11. "Postmenopausal women suffer bone loss with SSRIs," presented at meeting of the American Society of Bone and Mineral Research, Oct 2004, Seattle, WA.

6. Meijer WE, Heerdink ER, Nolen WA, et al., "Association of risk of abnormal bleeding with degree of serotonin reuptake inhibition by

antidepressants," *Archives of Internal Medicine* 2004 Nov 22; 164 (21): 2367–70.

7. Motl RW, Birnbaum AS, Kubik MY, Dishaman RK, "Naturally occurring changes in physical activity are inversely related to depressive symptoms during early adolescence," *Psychosomatic Medicine* 2004 May–Jun; 66 (3): 336–42.

8. Dunn AL, Trivedi MH, Kampert JB, Clark CG, Chambliss HO, "Exercise treatment for depression: efficacy and dose response," *American Journal of Preventive Medicine* 2005 Jan; 28 (1): 140–1.

9. Babyak M, Blumenthal JA, Herman S, Khatri P, Dorsaiswamy M, Moore K, Craighead WE, Baldewicz TT, Krishnan KR, "Exercise treatment for major depression: maintenance of therapeutic benefit at 10 months," *Psychosomatic Medicine* 2000 Sep–Oct; 62 (5): 633–38.

10. LeTourneau M, "Pump Up to Cheer Up," *Psychology Today* May–June 2001.

11. Bruder GE, Stewart JW, Tenke CE, et al., "Electroencephalographic and perceptual asymmetry differences between responders and nonresponders to an SSRI antidepressant," *Biology and Psychiatry* 2001 Mar 1; 49 (5): 416–25. Bruder GE, Stewart JW, McGrath PJ, et al., "Dichotic listening tests of functional brain asymmetry predict response to fluoxetine in depressed women and men," *Neuropsychopharmacology* 2004 Sep; 29 (9): 1752–61.

12. Ohara K, "Omega-3 fatty acids in mood disorders," *Seishin Shinkeigaku Zasshi* 2005; 107 (2): 118–26.

13. Vieth R, Kimball S, Hu A, Walfish PG, "Randomized comparison of the effects of the vitamin D_3 adequate intake versus 100 mcg (4,000 IU) per day on biochemical responses and the wellbeing of patients," *Nutrition Journal* 2004 Jul 19; 3 (1): 8.

14. Gastpar M, Singer A, Zeller K, "Efficacy and tolerability of *Hypericum* extract STW3 in long-term treatment with a once-daily dosage in comparison with sertraline," *Pharmacopsychiatry* 2005 Mar; 38 (2): 78–86. Szegedi A, Kohnen R, Dienel A, Kieser M, "Acute treatment of moderate to severe depression with *Hypericum* extract WS 5570 (St.

John's wort): Randomised controlled double blind non-inferiority trial versus paroxetine," *British Medical Journal* 2005 Mar 5; 330 (7490): 503; e-pub 2005 Feb 11.

15. Alpert JE, Papakostas G, Mischoulon D, et al, "S-adenosyl-L-methionine (SAMe) as an adjunct for resistant major depressive disorder: An open trial following partial or nonresponse to selective serotonin reuptake inhibitors or venlafaxine," *Journal of Clinical Psychopharmacology* 2004 Dec; 24 (6): 661–64.

16. Wilson VE, Peper E, "The effects of upright and slumped postures on the recall of positive and negative thoughts," *Applied Psychophysiology and Biofeedback* 2004 Sep; 29 (3): 189–95.

17. Ray US, Mukhopadhyaya S, Purkayastha SS, et al., "Effect of yogic exercises on physical and mental health of young fellowship course trainees," *Indian Journal of Physiology and Pharmacology* 2001 Jan; 45 (1): 37–53.

CHAPTER TWELVE: LISTENING TO MOTHER NATURE: ALTERNATIVE REMEDIES FOR OTHER HEARING PROBLEMS

1. Holstein N, "Ginkgo special extract EGb 761 in tinnitus therapy: An overview of results of completed clinical trials," *Fortschritte der Medizin Originalia* 2001 Jan 11; 118 (4): 157–64.

2. Sarrell EM, Cohen HA, Kahan E, "Naturopathic treatment for ear pain in children," *Pediatrics* 2003 May; 111 (5 pt 1): e574–79.

3. Wustrow TP; Otovowen Study Group, "Alternative versus conventional treatment strategy in uncomplicated acute otitis media in children: A prospective, open, controlled parallel-group comparison," *International Journal of Clinical Pharmacology Therapy* 2004 Feb; 42 (2): 110–19.

INDEX

described, 80
dosage, 87
synergy with ALA and ALC, 82–83,
    86–89
Colorado State University, 134
Columbia University, 201–202
common aging deletion, 30
    see also age-related hearing loss
completely-in-canal (CIC) hearing aids,
    218, 219
complex carbohydrates, 194
computer noise, 51
conductive hearing loss, 59–60
    hearing aids for, 217
Cooper Institute, 75
copper, 79
    described, 112
Cornell University, 146
coronary artery disease, 73
Corti, Alfonso, 17
cortisol, 193
Coumadin, 139
C-reactive protein, 75
Crestor, 62
cyanocobalamin, *see* Vitamin B$_{12}$

Deafness Research Foundation, 4
decibels (dB), 25–26
    earplug ratings in, 170–71
depression, 45, 84, 136, 193, 198–206
    diagnosis of, 198
    drugs to treat, 42–43, 44, 199–202
    easing feelings of, 206
    elderly victims of, 199–200
    fats and, 202–203
    hearing tests and, 201–202
    physical activity and, 200–201
    physical consequences of, 199
    SAM-e and, 200, 205–206
    St.-John's-wort and, 200, 205
    vitamin D and, 203–204
diabetes, 27, 45, 75, 84, 126, 131, 133,
    142, 193
Dietary Supplement Health and Education
    Act of 1994 (DSHEA), 104
dieting, 147
    dos and don'ts, 147–49

eggs and, 154–55
exercise and, 165–66
obsession with, 165
    see also moderation
diet strategy, 68, 69–70, 116–55
    better food equals better hearing,
        121–22
    BMI and, *see* body mass index (BMI)
    defining "healthy" weight, 120–21
    eggs and, 154–55
    good fats and, *see* fats, good
    guidelines for, 122–23
    how weight harms hearing, 119
    Mediterranean diet, 153–55
    moderation and, 146–50
    obesity epidemic and, 117–18
    starting point, 150–53
    sugar and corn syrup, 142–46, 149
    whole foods and, *see* whole foods
dining out, 146–47
distress, 193
DNA (deoxyribonucleic acid), 29, 39
    mitochondrial, 30–31
docosahexaenoic acid (DHA), 136–37,
    138, 194, 203
dopamine, 205
dried fruit, 134
*Drug-Induced Nutrient Depletion
    Handbook,* 76
drugs:
    decongestants, 179
    hearing loss and, 42–46, 52–53, 62–64
    -supplement interactions, 63
    see also specific drugs
Duke University, 201

ear, nose, and throat (ENT) doctors, *see*
    hearing professionals
    ear canal, 13
    hearing aids and, 218, 219, 221
eardrum, 15, 16
    air pressure and, 21
    rupture of, 64
ear infections, 21–22
    alternative remedies for, 210–11
ear protection, 68, 71, 169–81
    earmuffs, 173

ABOUT THE AUTHORS

Michael D. Seidman, MD, FACS, is a leading research physician in the field of otolaryngology with both undergraduate and medical degrees from the University of Michigan. Dr. Seidman is the director of the Division of Otologic/Neurotologic Surgery in the Department of Otolaryngology-Head and Neck Surgery, director of the Otology Research Laboratory, co-director of the Tinnitus Center, and chair of the Complementary/Integrative Medicine Program at Henry Ford Health Systems. He is the founder and CEO of Body Language Vitamin Co. and serves as a consultant for several teams in the NHL, NFL, and the ABA. He lives with his wife and three children in Michigan.

Marie Moneysmith is the author of *The User's Guide to Good Fats and Bad Fats* and *The User's Guide to Carnosine* and coauthor of *The User's Guide to Cartenoids and Flavonoids*. She is articles' editor for *Great Life* magazine and a contributing editor for *Let's Live*. Her feature stories have also appeared in *Better Nutrition,* the *Los Angeles Times, LA Style, Angeles, Home,* and worth.com.

NOTES

NOTES

NOTES